A Critical History of Dementia Studies

This book offers the first ever critical history of dementia studies.

Focusing on the emergence of dementia studies as a discrete area of academic interest in the late 20th and early 21st centuries, it draws on critical theory to interrogate the very notion of dementia studies as an entity, shedding light on the affinities and contradictions that characterise the field. Drawing together a collection of internationally renowned experts in a variety of fields, including people with dementia, this volume includes perspectives from education, the arts, human rights and much more. This critical history sets out the shared intellectual space of 'dementia studies', from which non-medical dementia research can progress.

The book is intended for researchers, academics and students of dementia studies, social gerontology, disability, chronic illness, health and social care. It will also appeal to activists and practitioners engaged in social work and caregiving involved in dementia research.

James Rupert Fletcher is a Wellcome fellow in the Department of Sociology at the University of Manchester, UK. His research covers several areas of the dementia economy, with an emphasis on using social theory and methods to understand dementia as a political entity. He has published on subjects including informal dementia care networks, mental capacity legislation and its influence on research governance, the anti-ageing technoscience market, anti-stigma and awareness raising campaigns regarding psychiatric disorder, the operationalisation of ethnicity and age in research, the biomarker discovery economy, the curation of dementia-friendly cultural events, dementia prevention public health strategies and environmental effects on cognition in urban settings. His lecturing spans medical sociology, the sociology of ageing, social research methods and ethical governance.

Andrea Capstick is an associate professor at the University of Bradford School of Dementia Studies. She originally worked alongside the late Professor Tom Kitwood to develop the first distance learning programme in dementia studies. Since then, she has at different times led both the BSc (Hons) and the MSc programmes in dementia studies at the University of Bradford. She holds a Doctorate in Education (EdD) for her work on the use of film and narrative biography in teaching dementia studies, and has published on a variety of subjects including participatory visual methods, arts-based approaches to teaching and learning, the representation of people with dementia in the popular media and dementia as a human rights issue. She has undertaken research funded by the NIHR (2012–15) on the impact of participatory filmmaking on social inclusion and well-being for people with dementia in long-term care, and more recently on the study 'What works in dementia education and training?' (2015–18) where she led the Patient and Public Involvement (PPI) work.

Dementia in Critical Dialogue

This series will bring together diverse and multidisciplinary commentators around key areas for development in the field of dementia studies. It will include, but not be restricted to, edited collections and monographs that will embrace a dialogic and relational approach where writers from within the field of dementia studies engage in a critical exchange with those from other fields.

The series will offer a critical perspective on key and emerging issues for the field of dementia with relevance to research, policy and practice. It contains a reasonable mix of theoretical, policy-related, methodological and applied research contributions. We would like to encourage texts that incorporate transnational and majority world/Global South perspectives in the understanding of dementia. The series editors will appoint a volume editor(s) and work closely with them to help bring together an appropriate mix of authors for each edition.

Series Editors:
Richard Ward (richard.ward1@stir.ac.uk)
Linn J. Sandberg (linn.sandberg@sh.se)
James Fletcher (james.fletcher@manchester.ac.uk)
Andrea Capstick (A.J.Capstick@bradford.ac.uk)

If you wish to submit a book proposal for the series, please contact the Series Editors or Emily Briggs emily.briggs@tandf.co.uk

Critical Dementia Studies
An Introduction
Edited by Richard Ward and Linn J. Sandberg

For more information on the series, please visit: https://www.routledge.com/
Dementia-in-Critical-Dialogue/book-series/DCD

A Critical History of Dementia Studies

Edited by James Rupert Fletcher and Andrea Capstick

Routledge
Taylor & Francis Group

LONDON AND NEW YORK

First published 2024
by Routledge
4 Park Square, Milton Park, Abingdon, Oxon OX14 4RN

and by Routledge
605 Third Avenue, New York, NY 10158

Routledge is an imprint of the Taylor & Francis Group, an informa business

British Library Cataloguing-in-Publication Data
A catalogue record for this book is available from the British Library

Library of Congress Cataloging-in-Publication Data
Names: Fletcher, James Rupert, editor. | Capstick, Andrea, editor.
Title: A critical history of dementia studies / edited by James Rupert Fletcher and Andrea Capstick.
Description: Abingdon, Oxon ; New York, NY : Routledge, 2024. | Series: Dementia in critical dialogue | Includes bibliographical references and index.
Identifiers: LCCN 2023014428 (print) | LCCN 2023014429 (ebook) | ISBN 9781032268774 (hardback) | ISBN 9781032268828 (paperback) | ISBN 9781003290353 (ebook)
Subjects: LCSH: Dementia--Research.
Classification: LCC RC521 .C756 2024 (print) | LCC RC521 (ebook) | DDC 616.8/310072--dc23/eng/20230623
LC record available at https://lccn.loc.gov/2023014428
LC ebook record available at https://lccn.loc.gov/2023014429

ISBN: 978-1-032-26877-4 (hbk)
ISBN: 978-1-032-26882-8 (pbk)
ISBN: 978-1-003-29035-3 (ebk)

DOI: 10.4324/9781003290353

Typeset in Times New Roman
by KnowledgeWorks Global Ltd.

Contents

List of illustrations

Figure

Table

Contributors

Michael Andrews is a person with posterior cortical atrophy dementia.

Ruth Bartlett is an associate professor in the School of Health Sciences, University of Southampton and a professor in health studies at VID Specialized University, Oslo. Ruth's research and teaching interests are crosscutting, involving persons living with a dementia, citizenship, ageing, disability and inclusive methodologies.

Allison Batchelor is living with Alzheimer's.

Jacqui Bingham was born in South Africa and is now living in Stockport, Greater Manchester. She was a funeral arranger for 12 years, but was diagnosed with young onset Alzheimer's in 2018. She is an artist and researcher.

Paula Brown has provided facilitation services to the Scottish Dementia Alumni since 2019 and has worked on award winning projects in the field of dementia since 2004.

Andrea Capstick is an associate professor in the Centre for Applied Dementia Studies at the University of Bradford, United Kingdom. She teaches for the MSc Advanced Dementia Studies and her research interests centre on participatory visual methods, patient and public involvement and arts-based approaches.

Teresa Davies (AKA **Dory**) I was diagnosed with Alzheimer's at the age of 59 and later with vascular dementia. I am still me and refuse to be defined by dementia.

Robyn Dowlen is a researcher and evaluator working in the broad field of creative health, with particular specialism in the role of music in the lives of people with dementia. As part of this work, she has a strong interest in conceptualising and understanding 'in the moment' experiences and its relationship to creative arts participation. Robyn is a chartered psychologist and musician, and is chair of the British Society of Gerontology's Creative Ageing Special Interest Group.

Ronald Ferguson aka **Ronald Amanze**
In respect of myself I'm not a sufferer
In factor I still feel enthusiastic about life
And future prospects

(like an invincible archives)
Following an Alzheimer's diagnosis and once I over came all the assumptions
And the challenges of navigating social services ETC
It was Especially after a met the dementia diarist
I work up to a new reality
That there's so much more to life than just taking medication
And being encouraged to basically give up on life
I've learned to fly
I also learned the Art of talking up for myself
And being badly behaved

Rebecka Fleetwood-Smith is a creative researcher with a background in textile design and psychology. She specialises in designing creative, sensory and embodied research methods and has carried out research with children, young people, older adults and people living with dementia. Her work is predominately based in health/social-care settings and involves exploring ways to reimagine and enhance such environments.

James Rupert Fletcher is a Wellcome fellow in the Department of sociology at the University of Manchester. His research spans informal care, mental capacity legislation, anti-ageing technoscience, anti-stigma and awareness campaigns, operationalisations of ethnicity and age, biomarker discovery, dementia-friendly cultural events, dementia prevention and environmental effects on cognition. Before joining the University of Manchester, James lectured in the Department of Global Health and Social Medicine at King's College London, covering medical sociology, the sociology of ageing, social research methods and procedural ethics.

Heike Hartung is an independent scholar who has earned her PhD in English Studies from the Freie Universität Berlin and her PhD habil. from the University of Potsdam, Germany. In her publications, she applies the methods of literary theory and cultural studies to the interdisciplinary fields of ageing, disability and gender studies. Recent publications include the monograph *Ageing, Gender and Illness in Anglophone Literature: Narrating the Bildungsroman* (2016) and the co-edited collection *Ageing Masculinities, Alzheimer's and Dementia Narratives* (2022). She is a founding member of ENAS and co-editor of the Aging Studies publication series with Transcript, Bielefeld.

Julie Hayden is a person with young onset dementia, possibly Alzheimer's type, but first and foremost a person.

Agnes Houston was diagnosed with early onset Alzheimer's dementia, in 2006, at the age of 57. She is an active member of the Scottish Dementia Working Group. In 2012, she was elected vice chair of the European Working Group Person with Dementia, and is also a board member of the newly formed Dementia Alliance International. She has campaigned for best practice and improving lives of people with dementia especially sensory issues and dementia. She received a lifetime achievement award by Alzheimer Scotland in 2013. In 2015, she was awarded a member of the British Empire. She has also been awarded a Winston Churchill fellowship to develop work on the sensory challenges experienced by people with dementia.

Nick Jenkins is a senior lecturer in sociology at the University of the West of Scotland. Since 2014, he has been exploring posthumanist, multi-species and post-qualitative approaches to understanding dementia. Alongside his colleagues, Dr Anna Jack Waugh and Dr Louise Ritchie, Nick convenes the *Multi-Species Dementia International Research Network* (https://multispeciesdementia.org/). Established in October 2019, the network seeks to advance more-than-human ways of responding to dementia. Nick is the lead editor for a book to be published by Bristol University Policy Press in 2023, entitled *Multi-Species Dementia Studies: Towards an Interdisciplinary Approach.*

John Keady is a professor of Mental Health Nursing and Older People at the University of Manchester where he holds a joint position between the University and Greater Manchester Mental Health NHS Foundation Trust. John leads the inter-disciplinary Dementia and Ageing Research Team and was founding and co-editor of the Sage journal *Dementia: The International Journal of Social Research and Practice* between 2002 and 2018. He is currently a senior fellow at the NIHR School for Social Care Research, Manchester. His most recent authored book (with Emmanuel Tsekleves, Lancaster University; 2021) is titled *Design for People Living with Dementia: Interactions and Innovations* and is available through Routledge publishers.

Jackie Kindell is a speech and language therapist and is currently Head of Allied Health Professionals and Social Workers at Pennine Care NHS Foundation Trust. Jackie has worked clinically in the National Health Service for over 30 years specialising in the communication needs of people with dementia, working closely with those living with dementia and their family and friends. She has a particular research interest in rarer dementias that present with changes in language and has published in this area including exploring how life story work might be used creatively to support interaction in semantic dementia.

Gerald King is living with dementia.

Ana Koncul is a postdoctoral research fellow in health studies at VID Specialized University in Oslo, Norway. Her current research is focused on dementia, welfare technologies and universal design. Ana holds a PhD from the University of South-Eastern Norway and an MA in Semiotics (University of Tartu, Estonia). Previously, she was a visiting researcher at the Department of Media, Communication and Cultural Studies (Goldsmiths, University of London) and the Faculty of Health, Medicine and Life Sciences.

Ann Therese Lotherington is a professor of sociology at the Centre for Women's and Gender Research at UiT, the Arctic University of Norway. Her work explores ways we can live together despite differences in age, gender, ability, nationality, ethnicity and/or other differentiating mechanisms. Questions about how we can promote interaction and integration in society without standardizing ways of living are central. These issues are particularly urgent for individuals and groups of people who do not have or will not be able to live up to a given standard. In her current research, she works with people living with dementia and asks how everyday life can be organised to ensure that their potential contributions to societal development are actualised and their citizenship maintained. She does this by investigating inter-action and intra-action through creative processes and artistic activity. The methodological approach is qualitative art-based research, while she theoretically applies feminist posthumanist theory and citizenship theory.

Katherine Ludwin is a qualitative researcher whose work is particularly focused on ethnographic enquiry in the context of experiences related to dementia. She is interested in norms connected to family and intimate life and how those manifest in popular culture.

Clare Mason is a dementia care trainer and the Experts by Experience Lead in the Centre for Applied Dementia Studies at the University of Bradford. She works with people living with dementia and their families to develop dementia training, research and education. She delivers all aspects of dementia-care training to staff from dementia care homes, hospitals, hospices and other areas of the care workforce. She also delivers training in two observational framework tools, Dementia Care Mapping and SOFI (Short Observational Framework for Inspection). Prior to joining the Centre for Applied Dementia Studies, she was dementia support manager and UK dementia trainer for the Alzheimer's Society, based in Bradford. She also leads the Pathways Young Onset Dementia support group as a volunteer.

Nancy McAdam is a person living with dementia in remote and rural Scotland. She has been active in advocating for people living with dementia for the past 15 years. She was an early member of the Scottish Dementia Working Group, a founding member of the ECREDibles and is currently a member of the Scottish Dementia Alumni. She has been awarded a British Empire Medal for services to dementia and recently contributed to the book *Remote and Rural Dementia Care*.

James McKillop is a key figure – indeed the 'father figure' – in the development of dementia activism in Scotland. He has been living with dementia for over two decades and is the founding member of the Scottish Dementia Working Group in 2002. This is a group run by and for, people living with dementia. This is believed to be the first in the world, and has since been replicated, worldwide. James, now 82 years old, is struggling with the natural deterioration of his dementia, and the health problems, old age brings. But, he keeps going, as best he can, within his current capabilities.

Wendy Mitchell was diagnosed with mixed dementia and is now the proud author of two Sunday Times bestselling books.

Elizabeth George Onyedikachi is a doctoral research fellow at the Health Faculty at VID Specialized University in Oslo, Norway. Her project is focused on dementia, everyday citizenship and religio-culture in rural Nigeria. Elizabeth is a social worker and researcher whose work focuses on amplifying the voices and improving the wellbeing of people in vulnerable situations.

Martin Robertson is living with Posterior Cortical Atrophy (PCA). He lives with his wife and dog 25 miles outside of Aberdeen. He is isolated in his rural location, but also by his difficulties living with PCA. He is, however, making sure that he is still involved and finding opportunities to have a voice. Martin is a member of the virtual Scotland DEEP network and the Scottish Dementia Alumni. He is also a founding member of the ECREDibles research group.

Moïse Roche is a researcher in dementia, ageing and ethnicity at University College London in the Division of Psychiatry, UK.

Aagje Swinnen is a professor in Aging Studies at Maastricht University (NL). She has published on representations of ageing in literature, photography and film; literary approaches in dementia care; and ways in which artists give meaning to creativity in the later stages of their career. Her work has been published in *Journal of Aging Studies*, *The Gerontologist, Dementia, Ageing & Society*, and *Feminist Media Studies*. Her co-edited work includes *Popularizing Dementia* (with M. Schweda, 2015). Swinnen is the co-founder of the European Network in Aging Studies and co-editor of *Age, Culture, Humanities*.

Toby Williamson is an independent health and social care consultant and works in dementia research, education, policy and service development. For ten years, he was Head of Later Life at the Mental Health Foundation, a UK social research and development charity where he led a number of projects focusing on people's lived experiences of dementia and issues of equality, diversity and inclusion.

Maria Zubair is a sociologist, currently working within the Social Science, Applied Healthcare and Improvement (SAPPHIRE) research group at the University of Leicester, UK. Following a PhD in Sociology, Maria began her post-doctoral research journey in social gerontology working within an ESRC-funded New Dynamics of Ageing project. Maria's research has focussed primarily in the fields of ageing, dementia, health & care and ethnicity. Her current research interests fall broadly within the areas of social identities, diversities and inequalities in old age. This includes a particular focus on: social constructions of old age, ageing and health; ageing and later life among racialised/minoritised ethnic groups; 'race'/racialisation within public health discourses; intersectionality, negotiation and performativity of social identities; social relationships and support networks in old age; health and social care provision for older populations; and gendered experiences of ageing, later life and health and wellbeing.

Acknowledgements

James Fletcher and Andrea Capstick jointly developed this book project, building upon a series of face-to-face and online workshops of the Critical Dementia Studies Network. The network was co-founded by Richard Ward and Linn Sandberg and supported through funding secured by Sandberg from Forte: The Swedish Research Council for Health, Working Life and Welfare (Grant nr Dnr. F18-1231-1). The editors wish to thank the funders, Ward and Sandberg, and all the members of the Critical Dementia Network for making the workshops such stimulating and educative events. An equal editorial contribution to this book was made by the editors.

Introduction

Andrea Capstick and James Rupert Fletcher

The first volume in this series (Ward and Sandberg, 2023) concluded with a rejection of any sort of 'big bang' account of dementia scholarship (critical or otherwise) characterised by sudden flashes of inspiration or paradigm shifts. Instead, Ward and Sandberg emphasise a need for iteratively re-working the genesis of dementia and dementia studies as transient, multiple and often contradictory political entities. This second volume extends that argument, applying the same approach to the recent history of social scientific and humanities scholarship regarding dementia. Hence, the chapters within it aim to shed light on some of the perturbations through which the material described in the first volume has come to be, in its contemporary forms. Rather than existing merely as 'the past'; that is, as an inert background to the present state of affairs, or what the critical philosopher Walter Benjamin (1940, trans. 1999: 154) refers to as 'homogeneous, empty time'. The history outlined in these pages can better be appreciated as a temporal politics with profound continuing influence.

It is often helpful for an introduction to start by defining key terms. In this case, we need to start by defining, first of all, what this book is *not*. It is not a 'history of dementia' (not even a critical one) nor is it an account of the development over time of dementia studies as a discipline, although it does include elements of both. The work of this volume is re-doubled in that it is a critical history of dementia studies. By this we mean that collectively these chapters offer an exploration and exegesis of some of the main trends in thinking around dementia in recent decades and particularly of ideas which are associated with the emergence of dementia studies as a distinct area of scholarship.

This has been a period which many working in the field associate with new waves of opinion, challenging what is often still described as the 'medical' or 'bio-medical' model of dementia (see Chapter 1 by Fletcher). The actual picture – as will become evident within this text – is more complicated, and one of our main purposes here is to avoid the exaggeratedly neat storyline often imposed on disciplinary histories. Instead, we hope to demonstrate trajectories that are more complex, overlapping and multi-dimensional. The history of dementia studies is not one of unilinear progress from an unenlightened past to an all-knowing present, but instead follows a circuitous and roundabout route characterised by repetitions,

DOI: 10.4324/9781003290353-1

elisions and blind spots. Our text correspondingly aims to trouble a widely accepted history in which dementia studies has moved from medicalisation to person-centred care to social citizenship and human rights-based approaches (HRBAs) with each of these 'lenses' representing progress over time. What we will try to show instead is that these different 'ways of seeing' dementia have often co-existed in various forms, and continue to exist as sets of overlapping and interpenetrating concepts, rather than as a sequence of historical 'stages'.

In many areas of the global North, this has also been an era of shifting allegiances and territorial disputes between academia and the practice field. The emergence of dementia studies as a discipline can in some ways be linked with contested views about the meaning and purpose of education, or of professional preparation, for working in the dementia field. In the United Kingdom, for example, the new relationship between the NHS and universities which accompanied the move of nurse training into higher education institutions (HEIs) raised questions about the content of curricula – about what, in effect, 'should be taught'. This move was accompanied on both sides by anxieties of influence (a term first used by Bloom, 1973 in the context of literary criticism). In other European countries, it is more usual for HEIs to specialise as either academically or professionally oriented. Nevertheless, European Union moves to create an all-graduate nursing workforce by 2010, as part of what was known as the Bologna Process, led to anxieties on both sides of the divide (Davies 2008).

Up to this point, dementia education had been an unproblematic matter of teaching practitioners-to-be about symptomatology, neurophysiology and pharmacology. With the entry into higher education, however, came more challenging considerations: might dementia be a social construct, for example; is it or is it not 'part of normal ageing'; does knowing about neuropathology really help, and if so what does it help with? The possibility of different models of dementia, and different 'lenses' for viewing the condition brought it closer to existing academic work in, for example, disability rights and critical psychology and, with this, the practice focus on 'care' for people with dementia began to shift to a set of broader theoretical and methodological considerations. In the United Kingdom, the first dedicated HE programmes related to dementia were still designated as courses in 'dementia care', but by the early C21 the transition to 'dementia studies' was already underway (see, for example, Downs et al. 2009). In the United States, by contrast much of the impetus for an emergent dementia studies arose from critiques of what has been termed 'the Alzheimer movement', with its increasingly commercialised focus on technological and pharmaceutical research related to prevention and cure (for examples of such critiques see Fox, 1989 or more recently Whitehouse, 2008, and Chapter 1, by Fletcher, in this book).

Of course, these tensions are far from resolved, and dementia remains, as it has throughout this whole period, a subject precariously balanced on a theory-practice fault line. On the one hand, dementia offers fascinating new avenues for theoretical development in academic cross-over fields in which it has barely featured as yet. Memory studies, philosophy of mind, and semiotics (the latter explored in Chapter 4 by Koncul and colleagues) come readily to mind, for example, as do various other contemporary areas of social theory such as post-structuralism or post-humanism, many of which are also touched upon in this volume (see, for example, Chapter 11 by Jenkins and Williamson). Simultaneously, however, in the arena of lived experience, dementia is also a condition which challenges all of us, with or without a diagnosis, to act and respond in various ways.

This points to a further key development in the period under investigation; the rise of dementia activism and self-advocacy. Dementia has come very late to the patient and public involvement table, following a long period when family members or representatives of related charities were often called upon to act as proxies. Again, these exclusionary practices have not completely died out, but they are widely regarded as less acceptable today, and when we are engaged in debates about the value of theory for exploring dementia and its implications, it is vital to take into account what people who are living with a diagnosis of dementia want to be done, or wish to happen.

Along with the shift toward self-advocacy and activism has come an increasing tendency to frame dementia in the contexts of disability rights and human rights more generally (Shakespeare et al. 2017; Cahill 2018). Here again, though, lies a conundrum of the kind that will frequently emerge in the chapters of this book. People living with dementia are not homogenised by their diagnosis, and do not all experience the condition in the same way, or want the same things. The chapters in this book that have been written and led by people living with dementia (Chapters 3 and 12) amply demonstrate not only the political common causes shared by those with a diagnosis but also that shades of opinion can vary significantly, even on the subjects such as acceptable and unacceptable terminology. People who choose to engage in dementia activism and advocacy may therefore not be typical of others with a diagnosis, and there are still many groups of people living with dementia whose voices we do not hear (people with late onset dementia, particularly older women, people from minoritised ethnic groups (see Chapter 8 by Roche and colleagues), working-class people, people who are homeless or on the margins of society for one reason or another, those with learning disabilities or other long-term physical or mental health conditions; the list goes on).

When the proposal for this text was accepted by the publishers, we were therefore hoping for a series of chapters which demonstrated, ideally individually, but even more so collectively, that trajectories within dementia studies are complex, that they may be either resonant or dissonant, and that they are both multi-dimensional and multi-directional. We were certainly not looking for unanimity, but we were hoping for a self-reflexive awareness on the part of authors that history is retrospectively viewed through a variety of lenses, and that critical histories are multiple, fluid and sometimes in tension with each other.

We were hoping for contributions on many of those areas that have been mentioned above as offering potential for further exploration (for example, gender, sexuality, ethnicity, social class – and the intersections between them – human rights, posthumanism, neurodiversity, embodiment, materiality, creative methodologies, advocacy and activism) and we were hoping to hear from authors who, above all, care about their subject area and want to raise standards of scholarship within it, just as much as they want people with and without a diagnosis of dementia to stand in solidarity with each other (two things which are, we would argue, ultimately inseparable).

Readers will judge for themselves how well (or otherwise) this has worked, and you may also wish to refer to the final chapter which includes our reflections on this subject as editors. Both as co-editors and as the authors of individual chapters within the text, we openly acknowledge we are, ourselves, part of the historical tradition the book seeks to deconstruct. All histories (this text included) are written under the influence of particular commitments, traditions and preconceived notions.

In that spirit, let us now move on to an overview of the contents of the text's 5 sections and the 12 chapters within them.

Section 1: Paradigms

The first section of this volume is titled Paradigms. Here, in two chapters which mirror each other in many ways, we challenge – as co-editors – certain sets of 'thought patterns' which have dominated dementia studies during the period in question. In Chapter 1, James Fletcher troubles longstanding critiques of the (bio) medical model in dementia studies. He advances an argument in favour of more biopolitical critiques, recognising the financial interests and power relationships that fuel the dementia economy, within which much dementia studies resides. As well as critiquing financialised biotech and charity alarmism, a biopolitical approach also requires a renewed attentiveness to dementia as a subjectivising political category, in reference to which citizens can self-govern in the interests of enhancing brain health, ensuring an active later life and limiting welfare requirements.

Andrea Capstick, in Chapter 2, critiques the ahistorical nature of much scholarship on dementia, and demonstrates how this focuses our attention on micro-social and psychological explanations of phenomena in the present day which may more properly be considered to have macro-social and political origins. This chapter holds that mainstream life history work tends to sanitise and conventionalise both individual life stories and the social histories within which they are embedded. This in turn has led to a significant lack of recognition of historical trauma among people now living with dementia, and along with this goes a failure to acknowledge the extent to which communal/institutional living can reactivate memories of past traumatic events. Finally, Capstick argues that we cannot usefully apply the concept of intersectionality in dementia studies without bringing a historical dimension to bear.

Section 2: Discourses

The second section, Discourses, includes three chapters, all of which, in various ways, examine the question of how language and thought are related in the construction of dementia. Chapter 3 – one of two chapters in this volume which have been contributed by people living with dementia – looks at the impact of terminology related to dementia which is often found in public discourse on those who are living with a diagnosis. Written by members of the Dementia Engagement and Empowerment (DEEP) group, the Pathways Young Onset Dementia Group, and the University of Bradford Centre for Applied Dementia Studies Experts by Experience Group with Clare Mason, this chapter presents a multi-faceted picture of the varying reactions of people living with dementia to these discursive elements. We hear how it feels to be on the receiving end not only of widely criticised terms such as 'dementia sufferer' and 'severe mental impairment' but also more innocent-sounding ones like 'living well' and 'dementia-friendly'. The material impact of some of these terms (for example, on eligibility for benefits) is also discussed, showing how such debates are not merely semantic.

The second chapter in this section, by Ana Koncul, Ruth Bartlett and Elizabeth George, continues this theme, albeit in a global context. The chapter demonstrates how pejorative terminology regarding dementia is embedded globally throughout many major languages. The authors provide detailed analyses of specific examples of negative terminology from a range of languages and discuss their implications for public awareness, as well as impact on those living with a diagnosis. Special consideration is given to those languages that do not have a word for dementia. It is, of course, difficult to establish why some terms are considered inherently more or less acceptable over time, with temporary shifts in acceptability in the name of 'political correctness' often not taking hold in the public imagination, or quickly being superseded by other favoured terms, so this chapter is also concerned with temporal shifts in acceptability of language.

Heike Hartung, in Chapter 5, attends to a different type of discourse; that of work in literary gerontology. Following a growing interest in recent years in pursuing understandings of dementia through cultural products, Hartung's chapter examines the connections between discourses of dementia from the 1980s onwards and the emergence of the dementia narrative. From early literary texts to the representation of dementia in one recent novel, *De Urolige* (2015; *Unquiet* 2019) by the Norwegian author Linn Ullmann, such products are used to outline a trajectory between medicalisation and diagnosis on the one hand, to more experiential and existential representations of dementia on the other. Ullmann's text is used as a case study – or paradigm example, we might say – for an alternative approach to dementia; one based on more creative, and potentially affirmative ways of engaging with forgetfulness. Taking such a cultural studies perspective, we are encouraged among other things to think about the potential connections between form and content, with experimental literary forms themselves offering insight into a world of spatial and temporal disruption, and of shifting discursive effects.

Section 3: Intersectionalities

Intersectionality is a term that has only recently begun to penetrate dementia studies. Coined initially by black feminists to capture the combined effects of misogyny and racism that were not experienced by their white counterparts, it is a term that has since been extended to also take account of such other 'dimensions of difference' as sexuality, disability and social class (see also Chapter 2, by Capstick, regarding the necessity of a historical dimension to intersectionality in dementia studies). Whilst intersectionality is a concept that applies par excellence in dementia studies, it also highlights a number of current blind spots in the discipline that are addressed by the three chapters in this section, on gender, ethnicity and heteronormativity, respectively.

In Chapter 6, Ann Lotherington examines the criticality of feminist approaches; not, it must immediately be said on the basis that women's experiences are to be privileged, but that such approaches have an inherent concern with inequality, oppression, discrimination and imbalances of power regardless of who is disadvantaged by them. As Lotherington acknowledges, however, feminist approaches have had relatively little to say about ageing or dementia, just as dementia studies has barely as yet engaged with feminist thought. Into this space, the chapter proposes three lines of inquiry that feminist approaches might offer to critical dementia studies; recognising dementia as a feminised field; applying intersectionality in dementia studies, and applying feminist posthumanist theory.

Chapter 7 turns to the equally 'new-to-dementia-studies' concept of heteronormativity. Here Katherine Ludwin examines another cultural product, the film *Still Alice* (based on the earlier novel by Lisa Genova) to draw out and critique a set of commonplace assumptions about the relationships, living conditions and family arrangements of people who have a dementia diagnosis. Such analyses help us to start unpacking overused concepts inherent in constant reference, for example, to 'people with dementia and their carers' or 'people with dementia and their families', which render invisible those who do not conform to heteronormative expectations regarding marriage, reproduction, and roles within families. As a result, Ludwin argues, there is an unspoken 'queering' of those who have never married, are childless, divorced, live in unorthodox households or are estranged from their families, in which sexual orientation, although one factor, is far from the full story.

In Chapter 8, Moïse Roche, Maria Zubair and James Fletcher focus on the contested roles of race and ethnicity in dementia studies. Taking the recent COVID-19 pandemic as their starting point, the authors demonstrate how predictions of illness risk based on race or ethnicity play into discourses which attempt to reduce health inequalities to individual genetic factors, lifestyle choices, or a combination of both. In this way problematic assumptions continue to be made about minoritised groups on the basis of presumed inherent deficits and essentialisation. The chapter provides a critical commentary on how such constructs continue to be allowed to stand in as biological and cultural explanations for health inequalities, thus supporting racialised discriminatory practices and perpetuating the view that reducing dementia risk is a matter of within-culture correction.

Section 4: Methodologies

Some of the most interesting developments in the last three decades in dementia studies relate to the active involvement of people living with dementia in research, education, practice development and public discourse. There are overlaps here, of course, with dementia activism and advocacy movements, but in the context of participatory research, for example, greater attention has been paid to the inclusion of people with a broader range of cognitive difficulties and abilities, and to the inclusion of people living with a dementia diagnosis who may not necessarily self-select to take part in public engagement. Inherent in this shift is the recognition, also, that traditional research methods are often not well-adapted to the preferences of people living with dementia. Bartlett and O'Connor (2010) point out for example, that orthodox 'sit-down' interviews are often not a pleasant experience for people with dementia, but this should create an agenda for the use of more creative methods, rather than for exclusion. Dementia studies therefore needs to shift from focussing on methods, per se, to a concern with methodologies more explicitly; that is to thinking about the principles and commitments which underpin the use of particular methods and approaches to creating data with people with a dementia diagnosis. This is a complex field, and it seems likely that a further volume in this series will be needed in order to do it justice. For the moment, however, this section includes two chapters on methodology, relating respectively to the use of life history methods, and arts-based approaches.

Chapter 9 is one of a number in this text (see also Chapter 3 by Mason and colleagues, and Chapter 11 by the Scottish Dementia Alumni) which were generated in a less-orthodox manner. Presented in the form of a dialogue between contributors whose work has previously taken them in somewhat different, although closely connected, directions, Jackie Kindell, Aagje Swinnen and John Keady's chapter is based on a transcribed online conversation about their differing conceptual and disciplinary experiences of life story work and the reasons for conducting it. The chapter reflects on the necessary entanglements and tensions inherent in life story work, its values and ethics, and on future directions in the authors' respective fields.

In Chapter 10, Rebecka Fleetwood-Smith and Robyn Dowlen examine the growth of arts- and culture-based approaches to dementia research in recent decades, which has not always been accompanied by a critical perspective. The authors begin by exploring the history of arts and culture in dementia studies. Providing an overview of the different theoretical positionings adopted by researchers when exploring the value of arts and cultural experiences for people living with dementia, the authors critically examine ways in which the medical model has permeated and continues to permeate arts and dementia research. Their appraisal examines the use of language, exploring historical and present-day literature to consider the ways in which dementia was and is framed and perceived and how this shapes engagement with arts and culture. They then go on to question the lack of reflection, over-reporting of positive outcomes and globalising assumptions about the extent to which arts-based approaches are enjoyed by people living with dementia which have tended to characterise this body of work.

Section 5: Politics

The final section consists of two chapters both of which touch, in interconnected ways, on the politics of dementia. The first, a debate between Nick Jenkins and Toby Williamson, focuses on the contested territories of human rights and posthumanism. Whilst acknowledging the importance of HRBAs, the chapter asks some interesting posthumanist questions about the potential for such approaches ultimately to play back into a form of liberal humanism. From a pro-HRBA position Williamson argues that such approaches can enhance the legal and social status of people with dementia and help counter images based on neediness and dependence. From a posthumanist, multi-species standpoint, Jenkins argues for a more radical project; one that is not dependent on human or cognitive exceptionalism. The authors conclude with some thoughts about how these contrasting perspectives can generate new debates in dementia studies as well as fostering social change.

Finally, in Chapter 12 members of the Scottish Dementia Alumni group, Agnes Houston, Nancy McAdam, James McKillop and Martin Robertson, reflect on several decades of personal activism in the shifting territory of dementia studies. After outlining the differing individual paths that brought them into campaigning in the first place, the Alumni discuss how much progress has really been made since the early days of dementia advocacy. This is a story of needing to shout long and loud in order to get a 'foot in the door' or a seat on a conference platform (a still-shocking account of being banned from one is included) in ways that many people living with dementia lack the resources to be able to do. On the ground, the authors note relatively little has changed, 'services are still limited and irregular, and a postcode lottery remains'. There could hardly be a more convincing way of underlining the text's rebuttal of the concept of linear progress over time than this final chapter.

* * *

We hope you will find the chapters which follow thought-provoking, and that you will encounter something new among them. Perhaps they will inspire, intrigue or annoy you enough to encourage you to write a chapter (or book) of your own as part of this ongoing series on Critical Dementia Studies.

References

Bartlett, R., & O'Connor, D. (2010). *Broadening the Dementia Debate: Towards Social Citizenship*. Bristol: Policy Press.

Benjamin, W. (1940). Theses on the philosophy of history. In *Illuminations* (1999 trans Zohn). London: Pimlico, 245–255.

Bloom, H. (1973). *The Anxiety of Influence: A Theory of Poetry*. New York: Oxford University Press.

Cahill, S. (2018). *Dementia and Human Rights*. Bristol: Policy Press.

Davies, R. (2008). The Bologna process: the quiet revolution in nursing higher education. *Nurse Education Today*, 28(8): 935–942.

Downs, M., Capstick, A., Baldwin, P. C., Surr, C. and Bruce, E. (2009). The role of higher education in transforming the quality of dementia care: dementia studies at the University of Bradford. *International Psychogeriatrics*, 21(1): S3–S15.

Fox, P. (1989). From senility to Alzheimer's disease; the rise of the Alzheimer's disease movement. *Milbank Quarterly*, 67 (1): 58–102.

Shakespeare, T., Zeilig, H. and Mittler, P. (2017). Rights in mind; Thinking differently about dementia and disability. *Dementia*, 18(3) https://doi.org/10.1177/1471301217701506

Ullmann, Linn (2020). *Unquiet*, transl. Thilo Reinhard, London: Penguin.

Ward R. and Sandberg L., eds. (2023). *Critical Dementia Studies: An Introduction*. London: Routledge.

Whitehouse, P. (2008). *The myth of Alzheimer's. What you aren't being told about today's most dreaded diagnosis*. New York: St. Martin's Press.

Part I
Paradigms

1 Pathologisation, (bio)medicalisation and biopolitics

James Rupert Fletcher

Introduction

In this chapter, I interrogate some of the conceptual bedrock upon which a substantial body of scholarship that falls under the moniker of dementia studies has been built. In particular, I focus on arguments regarding the (bio)medical model of dementia that have provoked significant criticism from social scientists since the late twentieth century, and which partly echo concerns from several decades earlier. While these anti-(bio)medicalisation critiques inspired influential dementia studies scholarship from the 1980s onwards, they were potentially already outdated. They attended to a version of dementia that, by that time, had been subsumed by something altogether different, that is, if that version had ever really existed at all. This dementia has little relation to (bio)medicine and has continued to evolve, especially in post-2008 political economies that create new speculative technoscience markets for capital accumulation.

Histories of dementia can often draw an unbroken straight line from the early twentieth century work of Alois Alzheimer through contemporary neuropsychiatric conceptualisations of dementia. However, this is a simplification that glosses over the suspect and relatively obscure nature[1] of mid-twentieth century dementia as an age-stratified disease. It also conceals the influential re-imaginings of dementia that flourished in the 1970s, and the important divergences from earlier orthodoxy, especially regarding ageing, both molecular and demographic. Here, then, I argue that we could benefit from disaggregating the neurophysiological pathologisation and biopolitical pathologisation of dementia as overlapping but meaningfully distinct phenomena, especially as the latter has manifested the peculiar biopolitics within which dementia studies are entangled. Ultimately, I argue that critical dementia studies could benefit from reconceptualising dominant imaginings of dementia in terms of biopolitics rather than (bio)medicine.

Neurophysiological pathologisation

The association between ageing, later life and mental deterioration has long been observed, stemming back to at least the Ancient Egyptians 4,000 years ago. Throughout much documented human history, the phenomena that we now consider

DOI: 10.4324/9781003290353-3

to constitute dementia have been understood as either a natural part of the human life cycle or a consequence of moral and/or spiritual weakness (Yang, Lee & Young 2016). Early efforts to designate dementia as a discrete and coherent psychopathological entity, in a manner that might be recognisable to us today, can be traced back to the work of nineteenth-century psychiatrists Pinel and Esquirol. They described a group of patients presenting with later life instances of broadly defined insanity and incapacity (Albert & Mildworf 1989; Boller & Forbes 1998). Importantly, this old age insanity was primarily conceptualised in terms of emotional pathology. This emotional pathology was unrelated to brain morphology and seemingly resided beneath what we might today consider the psychological, being more primal. It is now a rather provocative approach given the extent to which physiology has come to dominate mainstream institutional conceptualisations of dementia.

As general hypotheses of neuropathological nosology gained popularity throughout the nineteenth century, psychopathological entities were increasingly rearticulated in reference to neurophysiological vocabularies (Fox 1989). In this context, in 1864 Wilks wrote the first major neurophysiological description of dementia as a phenomenon rooted in observable brain atrophy (Wilks 1864). At the same time, as it was influencing psychiatric thought, the popularity of nosology also inspired biogerontological thinking on ageing as an amalgam of distinct physiological processes characterised by incremental degeneration and a range of associated diseases (Fox 1989). By the end of the nineteenth century, these two nosological trends were united in Binswanger's delineation of 'presenile dementia' in the under 60s and 'senile dementia' in the over 60s. The latter was normalised as an age-appropriate experience, while the former was pathological by virtue of its prematurity (Yang, Lee & Young 2016).

The abiotrophic delineation of presenile and senile dementias influenced what is probably the most well-known instance of dementia being pathologised, the early twentieth-century work of Alois Alzheimer with Auguste Deter. Alzheimer met Deter when she was sent to the Frankfurt asylum where he worked in 1901 with various familiar symptoms of dementia, including memory loss. Deter passed away five years later, and Alzheimer requested her brain for study. During this work, he observed atrophy, amyloid plaques and neurofibrillary tangles, the neuropathological hallmarks of the condition that now bears his name. Indeed, Alzheimer was renowned as a pioneering talent in microscopy development. Initially, his findings did not garner much interest among his peers, but in 1910, Emil Kraepelin elected to introduce 'Alzheimer's disease' into the eighth edition of his highly influential psychiatric textbook (Dahm 2006; Fukui 2015; Hippius & Neundörfer 2003).

In this early depiction, Alzheimer's disease was a discrete neuropsychiatric disease. It channelled Binswanger's distinction between presenility and senility to differentiate Alzheimer's disease from neurological and mental deterioration in later life and senile dementia. It is possible that neither Alzheimer nor Kraepelin was fully convinced by this age differentiation, with each articulating doubts to some extent (Beard 2016; Fox 1989). However, early twentieth-century Europe was characterised by fierce competition between laboratories to be the first to discover and classify new disease entities, particularly with Pick's institute in Prague and a wider range of psychoanalytic advocates. This likely provided some motivation for the two scholars to harden the conceptual boundaries of Alzheimer's disease and make it more fit for publication (Amaducci, Rocca & Schoenberg 1986). Hence, Kraepelin introduced the world to an Alzheimer's disease that was remarkably similar to senile dementia, but was different in at least as much as it occurred in people under the age of 60.

Perhaps unsurprisingly, the promotion of an Alzheimer's disease classification rendered meaningful by a patient's year of birth, and backed up with a handful of somewhat incoherent studies, was met with criticism (Barrett 1913; Fuller & Klopp 1912). At the time of publication, the neuropathological hallmarks that Alzheimer had documented were already recognised as being present in both presenile and senile dementias, as well as older people generally. They were generally considered to be too ubiquitous to be able to meaningfully demarcate particular disease classifications. Kraepelin approached this problem as one of degrees, whereby Alzheimer's disease was characterised by a significantly greater prevalence of hallmark pathophysiologies. However, this was, and indeed remains, a technically difficult claim to robustly evaluate given the difficulties of defining, isolating and reliably quantifying such neuroproteinopathies (Assal 2019).

In the early twentieth century, pathologists conducted detailed studies of the brains of people with dementia and determined that the proposed physiological characteristics of Alzheimer's disease were insufficiently distinctive to demarcate a discrete disease (Fletcher 2021a). In 1933, one post-mortem study reported neurofibrillary tangles and amyloid plaques in 80% of people aged 65 and above (Gellerstedt 1933, in Assal 2019). Nonetheless, Alzheimer's disease continued as a semi-accepted, if simply ignored, classification throughout the middle of the twentieth century. This persistence was not due to its clinical and scientific merit, but rather was attributable to the relative obscurity of the condition it described. By choosing to limit their dementia to younger people, Alzheimer and Kraepelin had effectively created a rare disease, because dementia is heavily associated with later life. Hence, Alzheimer's disease, while empirically suspect, was not subject to high-profile controversy by virtue of its epidemiological inconspicuousness (Fox 1989).

The physiological pathologisation of dementia created an interesting binary, couched in normative commitments to ageing and medical intervention. Presenile dementia was a distinct and rare pathophysiological affliction of middle age. Senile dementia was a nondescript and commonplace pseudo-natural experience of old age. This precarious schema rendered presenile and senile dementia unworthy of substantive attention, the former by virtue of its rarity, the latter because of its pseudo-naturality and hence inevitability. The conflation of dementia with ageing positioned it outside of what was generally considered the appropriate remit of medical interference (Beard 2016). Indeed, this is an issue that still constrains the acceptability of different forms of dementia intervention to this day. The normative inappropriateness of anti-ageing medical interventions is enshrined in contemporary pharmaceutical regulation because ageing is deliberatively not recognised as a valid indication by institutions such as the FDA and EMA (Fletcher 2020a).

While Alzheimer's disease remained a relatively unremarkable nosological entity throughout this time, insights into some of its purported neurophysiological characteristics were steadily developing with the aid of technological advances. For instance, electron microscopy allowed pathologists to explore cerebral matter from new perspectives in the mid-twentieth century. Some focussed on the neurofibrillary tangles and amyloid plaques that characterised Alzheimer's disease, producing publications that offered novel depictions of the suspect molecules (Kidd 1963; Terry 1963; Terry, Gonatas & Weiss 1964). The growing body of molecular evidence regarding these neuropathologies seemed to confirm what critics had long suspected, that if these were the hallmarks of a disease, then that disease was not pathophysiologically distinct from senile dementia. In hindsight, it can seem remarkable that this age differentiation of disease lasted as long as it did, but despite being radically transformed in the subsequent decade, senile dementia was not removed from the Diagnostic and Statistical Manual of Mental Disorders until 1994 (George, Whitehouse & Ballenger 2011).

Biopolitical pathologisation

By the 1970s, the neurophysiological pathologisation of dementia in reference to discrete cerebral characteristics had existed for several decades. However, the concentration of that pathologisation onto a group of people that rarely experienced dementia rendered it politically toothless. Hence, to become what it is today, dementia had to undergo a more politically astute pathologisation. This biopolitical pathologisation would hark back to and reinvigorated earlier physiological pathologisation by transforming its relations with ageing and the population to which it could be extended. As discussed, Binswanger's refraction of dementia through an abiotrophic binary of ageing versus pathology was not important enough to warrant high-profile critique. Nonetheless, it had been scientifically suspect since its inception, and the evidence against it had accrued steadily over the following decades. By the 1970s, research clearly showed that pathophysiological correlates with dementia did not respect chronological age cut-offs. However, as shown by Kraepelin's decision to publish Alzheimer's disease in 1910, evidence alone is neither sufficient nor necessary to transform dementia. Such transformation is political.

The biopolitical pathologisation of dementia, into a form that is familiar to us today, has been attributed to an Alzheimer's disease movement operating in the late twentieth-century United States (Arbogast, Welleford & Netting 2017; Chaufan et al 2012; Fox 1989). A key jumping off point in the genesis of this movement was the work of neurologist Robert Katzman, who united the physiological evidence on Alzheimer's disease neuropathology with epidemiological accounts of senile dementia. He noted that the age-based differentiation of presenile and senile dementia did not reflect pathophysiological or clinical differences, and that if those aged above 60 were included in the Alzheimer's category, then it was no longer a rare disease. Indeed, Katzman went so far as to claim that Alzheimer's disease was the fourth or fifth biggest killer in the United States (Katzman 1976).

As with most socio-political machinations, it is not entirely coincidental that Katzman turned to the epidemiology of senile dementia in the 1970s. This was a time when older people and population ageing more broadly were being intensified as political, and particularly fiscal, problems by virtue of purported implications for welfare expenditure amidst global economic crises. Growing demographic alarmism, articulated via 'rising tide' metaphors that echoed earlier racist rhetoric (Capstick 2011; Ineichen 1987), drew greater attention to statistical projections of age-stratified populations and welfare-relevant characteristics, such as age-associated morbidity. More older people meant more senile dementia. More senile dementia meant more public spending. Fiscal concern was echoed in moral panic regarding social reproduction, particularly fears of family disintegration and its implications for care. At the same time, again without coincidence, the National Institute on Aging was founded in the United States. Demographic alarmism bolstered the NIA's rationale, but associated political economic pressures also presented barriers to its development. Several stakeholders contested the NIAs creation on the grounds that there were already too many institutes, that the NIA would take resources from other institutes, that age-related issues were being addressed by other institutes and that ageing was technically and ethically beyond the scope of scientific intervention (Fox 1989).

In this context, the NIA had to fight for its survival. Key to this effort was the identification of an issue around which to organise, given that ageing as a general concern is rather nebulous and subject to intervention-scepticism. The NIA alighted on Katzman's de-aged Alzheimer's disease as a specific age-associated (bio)medical problem that could catalyse public attention and hence resources. To do so, the NIA established dedicated scientific conferences tasked with refining the problem and prospective means of addressing it, a funding stream focussing on the neurophysiology of ageing to encourage research interest, a grassroots advocacy organisation to coordinate government and public awareness campaigns involving people affected by dementia, and the forebear of today's Alzheimer's Association to organise high-profile fundraising and lobbying activities (Chaufan et al 2012). In response, the NIA federal budget grew 304% between 1976 and 1986, while its expenditure on Alzheimer's disease grew 2000% between 1976 and 1989 (Fox 1989; Kerin, Estes & Douglass 1989).

Throughout the 1970s and 1980s, NIA dedication to the promotion of Katzman's de-aged Alzheimer's disease rapidly generated a dementia that is familiar today (see Chapter 5, by Hartung, on the concurrent development of dementia-related literature during this period). Key stakeholders continue to endorse this dementia as *an age-associated cognitive syndrome with profoundly detrimental societal implications that is distinct from normal ageing and caused by various brain diseases that will be addressed through improved public awareness and technoscientific research enterprises.* While the physiological pathologisation of Alzheimer and Kraepelin is still embedded in this biopolitically pathologised dementia, it now extends far beyond their original concerns with a rare neuropsychiatric disease. This has been achieved by reconfiguring the relations between dementia and ageing. On the one hand, dementia has been de-aged, stripped of its age-segregated status and differentiated from 'normal' ageing. On the other hand, it has also been re-aged by bringing in later life cognitive decline, swelling the ranks of people affected by dementia and saturating dementia with the urgency of demographic alarmism. Somewhat ironically, as dementia has been reconfigured in relation to ageing, the earlier members of the category (those with young onset) have become increasingly estranged from it, despite remaining a core intellectual inspiration for aetiology and being at the forefront of institutional advocacy (see Fletcher 2021b).

Anti-(bio)Medicalisation

Dementia studies, in its contemporary iteration as a loose coalition of social scientific and humanities scholarships, emerged in dialogue with biopolitical pathologisation as it intensified in the late twentieth century. Drawing on a longstanding tradition of medical social science (Busfield 2017), early dementia studies scholars, e.g. Lyman (1989), Bond (1992) and Kitwood (1990), began to criticise the (bio) medicalisation and (bio)medical model of dementia. The core contention of their various arguments was that expanding (bio)medical classifications (e.g. dementia) were subsuming previously normal human experiences (e.g. cognitive ageing), and hence changing the nature of those experiences and the people affected by them. Paraphrasing Lyman's work, Spector and Orrell (2010: 957) define the (bio)medical model of dementia in a manner that will be familiar to contemporary dementia studies scholars:

> The medical model of dementia states that dementia is (a) pathological and individual, (b) organic in etiology (caused by progressive deterioration of those parts of the brain that control cognitive and behavioral functioning), and (c) treated and managed according to medical authority.

At face value, the observation that dementia has been (bio)medicalised is relatively obvious. Senile dementia was historically normalised in reference to ageing, and the Alzheimer's social movement contested that normalisation to make senile dementia a legitimate target for (bio)medical attention. By itself, this is not an explicit critique. However, the anti-(bio)medicalisation scholarship of early dementia studies did not stop at identifying classificatory shift. Critics were primarily concerned with the repercussions of those shifts for the people caught up in them. They argued that (bio)medicalisation extended unjust institutional power over people and devalued them by representing their experiences as pathological rather than meaningful. Both these phenomena are fundamentally dehumanising. (Bio)medicalisation permits the treatment of people within the category in a manner that is typically deemed unacceptable in relation to those outside of the category. Hence, it is dehumanisation owing to (bio)medicalisation, rather than (bio)medicalisation itself, that has historically provoked the ire of dementia studies (a legacy critiqued by Jenkins in Chapter 11).

The early psychosocial tradition of dementia studies was characterised by critiques targeting the dehumanisation of people with dementia as a result of the (bio)medical model influencing intersubjectivities. For Kitwood (1997) and Sabat (2001), the (bio)medical model fostered 'malignant social psychology' and 'malignant social positioning', respectively. In each instance, interpreting the person with dementia in line with the dominant (bio)medical model, led others to treat that person in dehumanising ways (see Chapter 3 for personal experiences of such treatment). In response, much work in the psychosocial tradition of dementia studies has attempted to rehumanise people with dementia, charting interpersonal methods for bolstering concepts of personhood, selfhood, etc., and hence pushing back against the dehumanising effects of (bio)medicalisation. The legacy of these arguments, advocating intersubjective rehumanisation in response to (bio)medical dehumanisation, remains today in an ongoing tradition of psychosocial scholarship (Fletcher 2020b).

As dementia studies scholars in the early twenty-first century began to question psychosocial preoccupations with intersubjectivity, the focal point of (bio)medical dehumanisation was retained. Critical dementia scholars, e.g. Bartlett and O'Connor (2007, 2010), began to critique earlier scholarship for depoliticising dementia. They argued that researchers who focussed on interactions were often problematically inattentive to the wider socio-political constitution of those interpersonal relations and of dementia itself. Important intellectual moves are made here. Personhood is replaced with citizenship, and interpersonal relations are replaced with socio-political relations (discussed further in Chapter 10 by Dowlen and Fletwood-Smith). What does not change is that (bio)medicalisation shapes the relations in question in a manner that leads those relations to undermine the person's status, in this instance his/her citizenship. Hence, despite notable conceptual theoretical divergences elsewhere, a critique of and challenge to (bio)medical dehumanisation is sustained across high-profile works in psychosocial and critical dementia studies.

Beyond work on citizenship, dementia studies' relatively recent turn to human rights has been similarly characterised by a politically sensitised approach, advocating rehumanisation in response to the (bio)medical model (Cahill 2020). Rights-based dementia studies have typically drawn on disability studies and the use of a social model in opposition to the (bio)medical model (Shakespeare, Zeilig & Mittler 2019). Again, this iteration of anti-(bio)medical argument has some important peculiarities, but retains many of the intellectual commitments that characterise the aforementioned areas of dementia scholarship. The (bio)medical model is still a focus of critique. It is still positioned as undermining the status of people with dementia, this time manifest in the person's rights. It is still judged to undermine this status because it constrains relations, this time the systemic relations that ensure those rights. In response, rights scholars advocate pushing back against the (bio)medical model, recognising that dementia is partially constituted within legal-political relations and can hence be targeted through policy and service provision (Cahill 2020) (see Chapter 12 for personal experiences of such changes).

Throughout the conceptual developments outlined above, the (bio)medical bogeyman continues to haunt dementia studies, often seeming to be a vague catch-all for the evils that dementia studies resists, from pharmaceutical profiteering to personal prejudice. Indeed, during the process of compiling this book, within which the question of what constitutes critical-ness is so pertinent, it became apparent that from one perspective dementia studies is inherently critical by virtue of its opposition to a (bio)medical model. Anti-(bio)medicalisation is a foundational orthodoxy of dementia studies, and it has been radically critical in certain respects, but the idea that it remains at the heart of critical thought on dementia is questionable. A mythic anti-(bio)medical criticality is potentially problematic when it blinds us to the extent to which the dominant model of dementia is actually far more biopolitical than (bio)medical, which has pronounced and potentially detrimental implications for people affected by dementia and dementia studies itself.

Biopolitical economy

There are several ways in which the dominant model of dementia (to the limited extent that such a thing can be said to exist) is not (bio)medical in a traditional sense. The argument that medical institutions and stakeholders enact undue control over dehumanised people with dementia is suspect in a political economy of care characterised by disengagement from healthcare services. The majority of people with dementia live outside of institutions with support from family and without formal medical interference (Fletcher 2019). Relatedly, the argument that (bio)medical stakeholders view people with dementia as disease entities is questionable. I have never met a geriatrician or psychiatrist who fails to appreciate dementia as a social experience formulated within micro- and macro-relational contexts. While such appreciation was less common historically, holistic understanding is now at the heart of these professions (Gawande 2015; Pollock 2021). In practice, austere political economic circumstances preclude holistic healthcare, but that is not necessarily a reflection of (bio)medical intellectual commitments or its practitioners. Similarly, the (bio)medical model has been critiqued for over-emphasising a pharmaceutical-heavy curative stance, but again, while political economic constraints may incentivise this, it is something of a strawman to claim that (bio)medicine is conceptually unconcerned with de-prescribing, prevention, rehabilitation, palliation, etc., an observation noted by several authors (Chaufan et al 2012; Leibing & Schicktanz 2020; Manthorpe & Iliffe 2016).

Outside of dementia studies, medical sociologists have long criticised (bio) medicalisation arguments as relatively outdated and blunt when it comes to understanding the contemporary influence of notions of neuropsychiatric health and illness in public life. They note that a focus on (bio)medicalisation can divert our attention away from the political and economic processes that drive hegemonic thought styles, and blind us to the subtle and pervasive ways in which biopolitical claims about psychic disorder permeate public cultures (Rose 2007; Williams, Katz & Martin 2011). Echoing these arguments, I suggest that, rather than a (bio) medical model, the dementia that was generated in the late twentieth century, and its subsequent intensification within post-1970s political economies, can be more incisively interpreted as manifesting a biopolitics of dementia. By biopolitics, I refer to the organisation of human life through the proliferation of a conceptual schema that compels the self-governance of personal conduct to serve the interests of the stakeholders involved in generating and sustaining that biopolitics (Goodley 2018; Mitchell & Snyder 2015). I have characterised a basic biopolitical dementia as follows:

> A syndrome of cognitive decline caused by discrete neuropathologies that are distinct from ageing, and … not enough people are aware of this. Furthermore, because dementia is caused by disease, and biomedical sciences have cured some diseases, dementia is a technoscientific challenge that will be solved through technoscientific endeavours.
>
> (Fletcher & Maddock 2021: 3)

There are several important differences from what has traditionally been considered the (bio)medical model. Institutional (bio)medicine has been relatively uninvolved in the biopolitical pathologisation of dementia, which has instead been led by charities, research institutes, advocacy organisations, government bodies, media and increasingly financial speculators. Biopolitical appeals to the involvement of (bio)medicine are hence not so much a reflection of actual engagement with biological science and institutional medicine so much as they are a symbolic method of cloaking biopolitics in the more socially respectable garb of science and medicine. Despite nominal appeals to (bio)medicine, the biopolitics of dementia is actually marked by substantive divergences from molecular and clinical knowledge. As discussed in the opening section, it has long been noted that the apparent neuropathological hallmarks of discrete dementias are ubiquitous in older people irrespective of cognition. One study of the amyloid plaques described by Alzheimer found that only 10 brains among 2,332 sampled did not have depositions (Braak et al 2011). Beyond amyloid, around two-thirds of all people aged 80 and over have an additional cognition-impairing neuropathology, e.g. infarcts (Oh et al 2014). Hence, the claim that dementia stems from discrete brain diseases *is* biopolitical and *is not* scientific or medical if we take those entities at face value (Herrup 2021).

Related to this, as a gerontologist I am constantly surprised by the manner in which claims regarding 'normal' or 'natural' ageing litter communications regarding dementia, including within dementia studies itself. The biopolitical ideal of the neurocognitively pure older person is an economics-motivated fabrication. Again, it lacks grounding in scientific or clinical evidence. Generally speaking, older brains atrophy and cognition declines, echoing senescence throughout the ageing body, and the two phenomena are not neatly correlated across individuals (Oh et al 2014; Taylor 2016). Critical gerontology has long revealed that appeals to 'normality' in relation to ageing typically reflect the normative convictions of the stakeholders making those claims and how those stakeholders desire older people to be, as opposed to any essential characteristic of ageing itself. In the biopolitics of dementia, normal ageing is typically characterised in terms of functionality. Critical dementia studies should reflect on whose interests are best served by the imposition of productivist ideals of function onto ageing populations.

Given that biopolitics relies on conceptual schemas to inform self-governance, it is perhaps unsurprising that it is characterised by information provision. As early as the 1970s, the Alzheimer's social movement identified that raising public aware-ness of their cause would be essential if they were to succeed. Indeed, the NIA's founding director explicitly sought to make Alzheimer's a 'household word' (Fox 1989: 82). Following this tradition, major dementia charities focus considerable efforts on information provision, awareness raising, campaigning, etc., peddling biopolitical messaging to transform public thought. In the United Kingdom, overall local authority social care provision rose from 2018 onwards, reversing a decade of decline. However, this increase was made up entirely of information provision, while practical provision continued to decline (King's Fund 2022). Information is conducive to biopolitical governance because it conveys the requisite conceptual schema directly to the public. It is cheaper than service provision (at least in the short term) and seeks to make individuals more socially reproductive, lowering formal demand and hence resonating with austere political economics.

Nonetheless, the biopolitics of dementia is also productively financialising in certain respects, particularly following the 2008 financial crisis, after which capital accumulation has become a major political economic concern. In response, the contemporary biopolitics of dementia generates a large market for speculative in-vestment. As mentioned above, dementia R&D budgets grew precipitously through the late twentieth century, and this growth has continued apace. In the United King-dom, government research funding grew from £28million in 2009–10 to £83mil-lion in 2017–18, with the 2019 election-winning manifesto promising to double this amount (UK Parliament 2018). This pales in comparison to the NIA's $3.5bil-lion budget in 2020 (NIA 2020) and $3.1billion dedicated by the NIH to dementia research in 2021 (AIM n.d.). In 2013, G8 health ministers met for a dementia sum-mit in London and established the £250million Dementia Discovery Fund to invest in promising drug discovery projects (DDF n.d.). Those countries also set up their own concurrent schemes, such as the £290million Dementia Research Institutes in the UK (DRI 2021). Despite this substantial biotech-centred financialisation, the pharmaceutical outlook is bleak and the technologisation of care, e.g. telecare or robotics, is often beholden to an ethics of efficiency that is in tension with an ethics of care.

Dementia research bodies often claim poverty relative to other issues such as cancer (e.g. Benham-Hermetz 2022), but in absolute terms, the field has rapidly become lucrative. The financial wizardry of dementia biopolitics has been to am-plify demographic alarmism as both a forthcoming welfare crisis and a prospec-tive consumer market, the former dystopian vision accentuating the latter utopian alternative. This means that resources flow into promissory technoscience initia-tives that claim to offer large returns on investment, while welfare is reimagined as awareness, friendliness, and latterly as preventative lifestyle choices. There is a lot going on here, and such issues cannot be addressed by decades-old anti-(bio) medicalisation critiques of interpersonal, socio-political or legal dehumanisation. Instead, they require a dementia studies that is alert to contemporary biopolitics and its heterogenous implications for people affected by dementia, spanning the proliferation of 'friendliness', (mis)regulation of pharmaceutical development, the identity politics of 'living well' and many more complex issues.

Conclusion

Dementia studies has long been motivated by a strong sense that something is awry with the contemporary status of dementia. The adoption of psychosocial anti-(bio) medicalisation critiques in the late twentieth century was a vital catalyst for critiquing some of the neurophysiological pathologisation that had long characterised later life cognitive decline. However, it has proved limited in its capacity to fully comprehend, critique and create alternatives to the biopolitical pathologisation of dementia that generated the conditions within which dementia studies itself has flourished. In response, critical dementia studies could benefit from fostering a keener biopolitical attentiveness to imaginings of dementia that have little relation to science or medicine beyond cursory gestures, and much more to do with responsibilising welfare and financialising demographic ageing.

This is not simply a matter of dehumanisation under the influence of a (bio) medical model. It is a question of making of humans and their lives, both with and without dementia, into self-governing publics and marketplaces that serve a particular set of interests. Contemporary dementia support is increasingly bound up with correct awareness as a precursor to correct conduct, while its future is financialised as an opportunity for capital accumulation. These circumstances are far more vulnerable to a biopolitical analysis than a (bio)medicalisation approach. Such analysis requires an expansion of critique to post-2008 political economic relations, the financialisation of demographic ageing, the responsibilisation of welfare, the neuropsychiatrisation of human life, etc. It also warrants a greater turning back of critique onto dementia studies itself, its processes of resource accrual and the biopolitical commitments that it can perpetuate.

Note

1 In line with the biopolitics-critical stance that I argue for, I deliberately adopt a new materialist approach to the 'nature' of dementia as akin to its conceptualisations and vice versa, rather than drawing strict distinctions between what dementia is and what we think it is.

References

AIM. (n.d.) https://www.alzimpact.org.
Albert, M.L. & Mildworf, B. (1989). The concept of dementia. *Journal of Neurolinguistics*, 4, 301–308.
Amaducci, L.A., Rocca, W.A. & Schoenberg, B.S. (1986). Origin of the distinction between Alzheimer's disease and senile dementia: How history can clarify nosology. *Neurology*, 36(11), 1497–1497.
Arbogast, C.E., Welleford, E.A. & Netting, F.E. (2017). State dementia plans and the Alzheimer's disease movement: Framing diagnosis, prognosis, and motivation. *Journal of Applied Gerontology*, 36(7), 840–863.
Assal, F. (2019). History of dementia. *A History of Neuropsychology*, 44, 118–126.
Barrett, A.M. (1913). A case of Alzheimer's disease with unusual neurological disturbances. *The Journal of Nervous and Mental Disease*, 40, 361–374.

Bartlett, R. & O'Connor, D. (2007). From personhood to citizenship: Broadening the lens for dementia practice and research. *Journal of Aging Studies*, 21, 107–118.

Bartlett, R. & O'Connor, D. (2010). *Broadening the Dementia Debate: Towards Social Citizenship*. Bristol: Policy Press.

Beard, R.L. (2016). *Living with Alzheimer's: Managing Memory Loss, Identity, and Illness*. New York: New York University Press.

Benham-Hermetz, S. (2022). The Health Secretary's vision for cancer could be a blueprint for tackling dementia. https://www.alzheimersresearchuk.org/blog/the-health-secretarys-vision-for-cancer-could-be-a-blueprint-for-tackling-dementia/.

Boller, F. & Forbes, M.M. (1998). History of dementia and dementia in history: An overview. *Journal of the Neurological Sciences*, 158(2), 125–133.

Bond, J. (1992). The medicalization of dementia. *Journal of Aging Studies*, 6(4), 397–403.

Braak, H., Thal, D.R., Ghebremedhin, E. & Del Tredici, K. (2011). Stages of the pathologic process in Alzheimer disease: Age categories from 1 to 100 years. *Journal of Neuropathology & Experimental Neurology*, 70(11), 960–969.

Busfield, J. (2017). The concept of medicalisation reassessed. *Sociology of Health & Illness*, 39(5), 759–774.

Cahill, S. (2020). New analytical tools and frameworks to understand dementia: What can a human rights lens offer?. *Ageing & Society*. doi:10.1017/S0144686X20001506.

Capstick, A. (2011). Reducing senility to 'bare life'. In Lister, J. (ed.) *Europe's Health for Sale? The Heavy Cost of Privatization*. Faringdon: Libri.

Chaufan, C., Hollister, B., Nazareno, J. & Fox, P. (2012). Medical ideology as a double-edged sword: The politics of cure and care in the making of Alzheimer's disease. *Social Science & Medicine*, 24, 788–795.

Dahm, R. (2006). Alzheimer's discovery. *Current Biology*, 16(21), R906–R910.

DDF (n.d.) Dementia Discovery Fund. https://svhealthinvestors.com/funds/the-dementia-discovery-fund.

DRI (2021). Dementia Research Institutes. https://ukdri.ac.uk/about-us.

Fletcher, J.R. (2019). A methodological approach to accessing informal dementia care. *Working with Older People*, 23(4), 228–240.

Fletcher, J.R. (2020a). Anti-aging technoscience & the biologization of cumulative inequality: Affinities in the biopolitics of successful aging. *Journal of Aging Studies*, 55, 100899.

Fletcher, J.R. (2020b). Distributed selves: Shifting inequities of impression management in couples living with dementia. *Symbolic Interaction*, 43, 405–427.

Fletcher, J.R. (2021a). Black knowledges matter: How the suppression of non-white understandings of dementia harms us all and how we can combat it. *Sociology of Health & Illness*, 43(8), 1818–1825.

Fletcher, J.R. (2021b). Destigmatising dementia: The dangers of felt stigma and benevolent othering. *Dementia*, 20(2), 417–426.

Fletcher, J.R. & Maddock, C. (2021). Dissonant dementia: Neuropsychiatry, awareness, and contradictions in cognitive decline. *Humanities and Social Sciences Communications*, 8(1), 1–11.

Fox, P. (1989). From senility to Alzheimer's disease: the rise of the Alzheimer's disease movement. *The Milbank Quarterly*, 67, 58–102.

Fukui, T. (2015). Historical review of academic concepts of dementia in the world and Japan: With a short history of representative diseases. *Neurocase*, 21(3), 369–376.

Fuller, S.C. & Klopp, H.I. (1912). Further observations on Alzheimer's disease. *American Journal of Insanity*, 69(1), 17–29.

Gawande, A. (2015). *Being Mortal: Illness, Medicine and What Matters in the End*. London: Profile Books.

George, D.R., Whitehouse, P.J. & Ballenger, J. (2011). The evolving classification of dementia: Placing the DSM-V in a meaningful historical and cultural context and pondering the future of "Alzheimer's". *Culture, Medicine, and Psychiatry*, 35(3), 417–435.

Goodley, D. (2018). Understanding disability: Biopsychology, biopolitics, and an in-between-all politics. *Adapted Physical Activity Quarterly*, 35(3), 308–319.

Herrup, K. (2021). *How Not to Study a Disease: The Story of Alzheimer's*. Cambridge: MIT Press.

Hippius, H. & Neundörfer, G. (2003). The discovery of Alzheimer's disease. *Dialogues in Clinical Neuroscience*, 5(1), 101–108.

Ineichen, B. (1987). Measuring the rising tide: How many dementia cases will there be by 2001?. The *British Journal of Psychiatry*, 150(2), 193–200.

Katzman, R. (1976). The prevalence and malignancy of Alzheimer disease: A major killer. *Archives of Neurology*, 33(4), 217–218.

Kerin, P.B., Estes, C.L. & Douglass, E.B. (1989). Federal funding for aging education and research: A decade analysis. *The Gerontologist*, 29(5), 606–614.

Kidd, M. (1963). Paired helical filaments in electron microscopy of Alzheimer's disease. *Nature*, 197(4863), 192–193.

King's Fund. (2022). Social Care 360: Workforce and Carers. https://www.kingsfund.org.uk/publications/social-care-360/workforce-and-carers.

Kitwood, T.M. (1990). The dialectics of dementia: With particular reference to Alzheimer's disease. *Ageing & Society*, 10(2), 177–196.

Kitwood, T.M. (1997). *Dementia Reconsidered: The Person Comes First*. Buckingham: Open University Press.

Leibing, A. & Schicktanz, S. (Eds.). (2020). *Preventing Dementia?: Critical Perspectives on a New Paradigm of Preparing for Old Age*. New York: Berghahn Books.

Lyman, K.A. (1989). Bringing the social back in: A critique of the biomedicalization of dementia. *The Gerontologist*, 29(5), 597–605.

Manthorpe, J., & Iliffe, S. (2016). *The Dialectics of Dementia*. London: Social Care Workforce Research Unit.

Mitchell, D.T. & Snyder, S.L. (2015). *The Biopolitics of Disability: Neoliberalism, Ablenationalism, and Peripheral Embodiment*. Ann Arbor: University of Michigan Press.

NIA. (2020). September 2020 Director's Status Report. http://www.nia.nih.gov/about/naca/september-2020-directors-status-report.

Oh, H., Madison, C., Villeneuve, S., Markley, C. & Jagust, W.J. (2014). Association of gray matter atrophy with age, β-amyloid, and cognition in aging. *Cerebral Cortex*, 24(6), 1609–1618.

Pollock, L. (2021). *The Book About Getting Older*. London: Penguin.

Rose, N. (2007). Beyond medicalisation. *The Lancet*, 369(9562), 700–702.

Sabat, S.R. (2001). *The Experience of Alzheimer's Disease: Life Through a Tangled Veil*. Hoboken: Wiley.

Shakespeare, T., Zeilig, H. & Mittler, P. (2019). Rights in mind: Thinking differently about dementia and disability. *Dementia*, 18(3), 1075–1088.

Spector, A. & Orrell, M. (2010). Using a biopsychosocial model of dementia as a tool to guide clinical practice. *International Psychogeriatrics*, 22(6), 957–965.

Taylor, K. (2016). *The Fragile Brain: The Strange, Hopeful Science of Dementia*. Oxford: Oxford University Press.

Terry, R.D. (1963). The fine structure of neurofibrillary tangles in Alzheimer's disease. *Journal of Neuropathology & Experimental Neurology*, 22, 629–642.

Terry, R.D., Gonatas, N.K. & Weiss, M. (1964). Ultrastructural studies in Alzheimer's presenile dementia. *The American Journal of Pathology*, 44(2), 269–297.

UK Parliament. (2018). Question for Department of Health and Social Care. https://questions-statements.parliament.uk/written-questions/detail/2018-11-19/HL11541.

Wilks, S. (1864). Clinical notes on atrophy of the brain. *Journal of Mental Science*, 10, 381–392.

Williams, S.J., Katz, S. & Martin, P. (2011). Neuroscience and medicalisation: sociological reflections on memory, medicine and the brain. In Pickersgill, M. & Van Keulen, I. (eds.) *Sociological Reflections on the Neurosciences*. Bingley: Emerald.

Yang, H.D., Lee, S.B. & Young, L.D. (2016). History of Alzheimer's disease. *Dementia and Neurocognitive Disorders*, 15(4), 115–121.

2 The century without a war

Kitwood's concept of malignant social psychology and the need for historicisation in dementia studies

Andrea Capstick

Introduction

Despite the popularity of life history-based approaches in dementia practice (see Chapter 10 in this volume for some contemporary examples), there has been a surprising failure to engage with social, national and international history in dementia studies. In this chapter, I want to outline some of the consequences of a dehistoricised view of dementia, arguing that this leads to an impoverished concept of intersectionality, as this term has so far been applied in the dementia field, and a failure to recognise historical trauma as a factor impacting on the lived experience of many more people living with dementia than we might think.

The chapter considers the implications of taking a whole-life view of dementia which includes awareness not only of dimensions such as age, gender, ethnicity, sexuality and social class but also the grounding of individual lives in the actually prevailing social circumstances during their lifetime. In social sciences generally, and in gerontology specifically, the lifecourse is recognised as a central, albeit complex, concept (Alwin 2012). Taking a lifecourse perspective involves a recognition (at minimum) that the socio-economic conditions prevailing throughout a person's life, the periods of history they have lived through, and the impact of internalised social mores belonging to those periods are all important influences in later life. Smail (1993) critiques psychosocial explanations which cite proximal and synchronic influences (nearby and in the present) as the source of social ills, while overlooking those which are distal and diachronic (further away and longer ago). In taking a proximal and synchronic view, Smail suggests, we are led to believe that problems result from the 'right' or 'wrong' acts of individuals, rather than socio-economic inequalities and imbalances of power. In this chapter, I critique Kitwood's concepts of person-centred care and malignant social psychology for their ahistoricism; that is to say, for their lack of a socially and culturally grounded lifecourse perspective and for the resulting suggestion that dementia is, as Kitwood puts it, 'an existential crisis of a person … and indeed a crisis of *an interpersonal milieu* (Kitwood 1990a: 60).

In advancing this argument, I draw on illustrative material from my own qualitative research and from narrative biographical work undertaken as part of the Trebus Project (directed by David Clegg), which I was involved with for many years.

DOI: 10.4324/9781003290353-4

Between 2001 and 2016, well over a thousand narrative biographies of people with dementia were collected by the Trebus Project. Originally published in two anthologies *Ancient Mysteries* (Brown and Clegg 2007) and *Tell Mrs Mill Her Husband Is Still Dead* (Bryce et al 2010), several of these narratives were later broadcast on Radio 4, and are now available at https://soundcloud.com/david-clegg

The life stories of people living with dementia are often put into other people's words, even when these words are attributed to the person in question. This tends to homogenise lived experience so that it is palatable to others (as, for example, 'My mother died while I was only young'). The autobiographical narratives from the Trebus Project are strikingly different. They are uncensored, and told in a first-person voice which is very evidently the person's own. They often have a visceral quality which makes the true import of the words hard to ignore or dismiss ('Mum was ill off and on for a long while – tuberculosis – she lost her life's blood. Christmas would have been the last day I saw her alive'.) This material challenges mainstream thinking on the value of life history work, seeing it less as individual therapy than as an opportunity to learn from those who have borne witness to history as it happened.

Historical trauma and social amnesia

It is widely accepted that life history awareness is one of the key requirements for providing person-centred dementia services (some of the most frequent approaches and debates are discussed in Chapter 10). Yet often these histories, even when they are done well on their own terms, are surprisingly ahistorical. The UK Life Story Network website (https://www.elder.org/the-elder/your-life-your-story-your-care-personalised-care-life-story-network/) points outs that life story books made with people living with dementia are often used at their funerals. There are good reasons for this. The recorded elements of the person's story are those that their remaining family wish to be known. After my grandfather's funeral, I remember my brother remarking wryly that when the vicar confidently announced that his wife, who had predeceased him by just under a year, would be waiting for him in heaven, he didn't mention two other former wives who might have something to say about that. Funeral eulogies airbrush life stories to make them palatable to the living. Similarly left out of most mainstream life histories are divorce, infidelity, children born outside marriage, unofficial adoptions, crime, domestic abuse, unemployment, child neglect and a whole range of other aspects of the domestic sphere that have been commonplace during the lifetimes of those who now have dementia.

Why is this important? At a purely individual level, knowing what has happened to a person historically may shed a great deal of light on his or her reactions in the present day. For example, we might expect a person who has been subjected to brutal corporal punishment for wetting the bed as a schoolchild to have a more profound fear of incontinence in the context of dementia.

They'd come up behind you and Bang! Smack across the ears I remember Father Cundry, he used a leather strap on you – very hard to explain such cruelty. If you wet the bed they'd line up … and get the kids to come down carrying the wet mattresses.

(Michael, in Brown and Clegg 2007: 36)

Beyond this personal domestic sphere, however, there is also the broader domain of social, national and international history. People who now have dementia have lived through wars, been conscripted to involuntary military service (as we will see below, this continued in Britain long after 1945), evacuated, interned, bombed, made stateless, lost multiple family members, suffered various forms of discrimination, harassment and abuse, and experienced natural and manmade disasters of various kinds. Many of them may never have spoken of these experiences prior to the onset of dementia, but for various reasons (relative disinhibition, unfreezing of affect, or a simple desire to set the record straight) dementia often seems to unleash memories that have previously been kept under strict cognitive control (Capstick and Clegg 2013).

Few people now living with dementia will have escaped all 14 of the main types of trauma listed in widely used scales such as the following one from the Georgetown University Centre for Child and Human Development (Saad 2019).

1. Natural or manmade disasters
2. Forced displacement
3. War/terrorism/political violence
4. Victim of, or witness to, extreme personal or interpersonal violence
5. Traumatic grief or separation, e.g. loss of parents or siblings
6. System-induced trauma, e.g. forced removal from home or family
7. Sexual abuse or assault
8. Physical abuse or assault
9. Emotional abuse
10. Neglect
11. Serious accident or illness
12. Witness to domestic violence
13. Victim of or witness to community violence
14. School violence

Using these categories as codes, I have carried out my own mapping of many of the 47 stories told by people living with dementia in the Trebus Project anthology mentioned above, *Tell Mrs Mill Her Husband Is Still Dead* (Bryce et al 2010). I found that almost all of the contributors disclosed experience of at least one such trauma; with some revealing repeated instances of traumatic events. Key findings for the first five narrators featured in the book are given below. The numbers correspond to types of trauma identified in the Georgetown University Centre typology just listed:

Fia lived through war and revolution in Angola (3); one of her children died in infancy (5).
Eva was born in Germany. Her father shot himself dead during Hitler's rise to power (3/5); she also witnessed domestic violence between her grandparents (12).

Grace's father was admitted to an asylum where he died when she was a teenager (5). Her husband was killed on D-Day, just days before their son was born (3/5).

Mabel's mother died when she was five years old (5). During the Blitz she was evacuated from London to Luton (6) which was also bombed (3). Her brother was killed in a plane collision while on active service (3/5).

Aidan's mother died soon after his birth (5). He was sent to foster parents he didn't know (6). He was beaten regularly by teachers (14), and became partially sighted as a result of one of them kicking a ball in his face (8). His brother was murdered in a hammer attack and he had to identify the body (4/5). He witnessed police violence against protest marchers (13).

We might be tempted to think that the contributors to this anthology are unusual in some way, but my own qualitative research with people living with dementia had very similar findings. Among 10 people I worked with on a participatory film-making study (Capstick and Ludwin 2015), Frank's Catholic family had left Northern Ireland when he was 16 due to sectarian violence. Henry and Rita were both evacuated during the war. Eileen grew up in a children's home where she was neglected and abused. Nora remembered the Jarrow hunger marches (there is no category in the Georgetown typology for extreme poverty and deprivation, but there should be). Florence's young son had been killed in front of her when a building collapsed. A priest had been called to say the last rites over Rose's three week-old son because he was not expected to live; her husband, she said, was in the pub with another woman at the time (a 9, I would say).

Part of my argument is, then, that mainstream life histories are better to be regarded as censored testimonies. They are the sanitised, compliant narratives that are permitted to be disclosed in care home lounges and at subsequent funerals. Whilst there could, of course, be no complete 'true story' of any person's life, it is almost certainly in the gaps, elisions and erasures of these conventional life stories that the most significant events of someone's life will lie. Most significant, because they will be the events which still carry an emotional freight of shame, fear, anger or regret that a person living with dementia may have reduced ability to keep under control, particularly if their current lived experience is reminiscent in some way of a past trauma. These are the skeletons partners and other family members often want to keep firmly in the cupboard. Sons and daughters may often not even know they exist.

To give a specific example, recently I was part of a working group producing a report on Sex, gender and sexuality in the context of dementia (Gove et al 2022) and was sent a draft to review. It rightly mentioned the stigma which may still be associated with same-sex relationships in the minds of older people now living with dementia. I started to reflect that in the youth of many people who now have dementia, almost any kind of sexual activity – other than the straight, married, monogamous and unprotected kind – was stigmatised. Sex before marriage was forbidden, unmarried parenthood was an outrage, contraception was synonymous with promiscuity, and masturbation would lead to hairy palms and mental retardation. Of course, even at the time, people were well aware of societal double standards on subjects like these. Yet we rarely see reference to the impact of such mainstream social mores in any discussion of sexuality and dementia (Chapter 7, by Ludwin, offers a valuable exception, which also touches – in its discussion of heteronormativity – on the ways the 'ideal family' has been socially constructed as straight, white, middle-class, monogamous etc. to the exclusion of all other forms of domestic arrangement). There is too little consideration that when times change, attitudes that have been long-internalised may not follow suit.

Within the field of critical psychology, 'social amnesia' is a term coined by Jacoby (1996) in support of his view that society at large has 'lost its memory', and is therefore unable to come to terms with national histories characterised by violence, exploitation and abuse. Collective memory, Jacoby argues, has been conventionalised to elide painful truths. Social amnesia is evident everywhere in the field of dementia studies, but because those living with dementia are often regarded as unreliable narrators, much of what they say for themselves is often dismissed as invention or confusion, particularly by those who, due to age or ethnicity, do not share the same set of cultural references.

Yet, in dementia, recall for emotionally charged events which took place between approximately 5 and 30 years of age often remains intact when short-term memory becomes compromised. This is sometimes referred to as a 'reminiscence bump' (Thomsen and Berntsen 2008). Events society has collectively and collusively forgotten are, therefore, precisely those most likely to be remembered by people living with dementia. Yet conventional life story work carried out with those living with dementia frequently elides traumatic social and national events and forms of abuse or persecution that were common in their youth. As Kruger-Fürhoff et al (2021) have recently pointed out that dementia has become a common trope for representing elided violent pasts in film and literary fiction. As yet, however, the narratives of actual people with dementia on such subjects have been accorded less attention.

Frances, one of the Trebus narrators, talks repeatedly about a 'beautiful boy' and a 'burning man'. She recounts a horrific dream in which the burning man is wearing her own clothes, which are on fire. Without a historical perspective it would be easy to assume that Frances is hallucinating or talking about something seen in a film, perhaps. In reality, Frances was a radio broadcaster in what was then Czechoslovakia during the Prague Spring of 1968. There, she witnessed the 19-year-old student Jan Palach intentionally set himself on fire in protest at Czech capitulation to the Soviet invasion. 'Some parts of history', as Frances herself notes, 'are deliberately forgotten'.

Developing a historical consciousness in Dementia Studies is not an optional extra, but central to understanding. It is, I would argue, a better guide to understanding the things people living with dementia say and do in the present day than are Kitwood's concepts of malignant social psychology and personal detraction, where behaviour is understood to be a response to insults to personhood on the part of those providing care and services.

The problem with malignant social psychology

Proponents of the deficit-focused biomedical model of dementia are keen to emphasise memory loss as its central 'symptom', arising mainly, if not solely, from progressive, localised brain pathology. Altered or lost memories are thus pathologised at the individual level, whilst being left unexamined at a societal level. Yet, in Kitwood's person-centred, or psychosocial, model of dementia there is also a retreat from history, and an intellectual air-brushing of the seamier side of human existence which is out of keeping with the real conditions under which people now living with dementia grew up and came of age.

Kitwood's concept of malignant social psychology was advanced initially as part of his attempt to demonstrate that much of the deterioration that occurs in people living with dementia is not the result of neuropathology, but of insensitive or discriminatory treatment by others. Kitwood reconceptualised what are referred to, from a biomedical perspective, as 'challenging behaviours' as needs-related ill-being arising from insensitive treatment and social exclusion. In particular, he identified 17 types of 'personal detraction' (including mockery, treachery, overpowering, ignoring etc) which – when observed frequently in formal dementia care settings – could be taken to indicate the presence of a 'malignant social psychology' (Kitwood, 1997a: 46–47). This typology of personal detractions has become widely known and used in dementia care practice. Kitwood also described what he termed an 'involutionary spiral' of negative events which tend to occur following a diagnosis of dementia, which work to exacerbate cognitive decline.

A major problem with this line of argument, from a historical perspective, is that we are encouraged to assume that prior to the onset of dementia the person concerned had never experienced personal detractions or negative life events. The person's involutionary spiral is triggered by diagnosis, it is implied, following a previous life of uneventful 'normality'. The 'vignettes', as he terms them, which Kitwood constructs to represent life before dementia reinforce this de-historicised worldview. For example, Arthur who 'had been a highly respected member of the community and a pillar of his local church … now … often offends people with his foul language, and some care staff are afraid of him, because when they come close he often punches or bites them' (Kitwood 1997: 75). Such examples suggest that dementia is the sole tragedy disrupting a previously unremarkable life. Yet if we assume that Arthur has a real prototype among those people living with dementia Kitwood had encountered during the research underpinning *Dementia Reconsidered* he must have been born in the first half of the 20th century. If he was very lucky, he might have been too young for conscription in the first world war and too old in the second world war, but he could hardly have escaped living through that period of history altogether. He would be very likely to have lost friends or relatives to war, experienced bombing raids, rationing, shortages and the constant threat of occupation. If we re-construct the vignette so that Arthur was interned in a Japanese prison camp for several years, for example, this puts an entirely different construction on his behaviour in the present day.

It is not, of course, that Kitwood never mentions historical events of this nature, but when he does they become – in a rather deft conjuring act – mere metaphors for the experience of dementia. For example, Kitwood (1997a: 74) cites work carried out by Cheston (1996) with a man whose military service was in the Malayan jungle, and who spoke of 'the persistent advance of the vegetation and the constant battle to keep it back'. This is interpreted by Kitwood as 'a way for him to talk about his *own* struggle with dementia' (Kitwood 1997: 74, emphasis added). Referring to the man's '*own* struggle with dementia' suggests a radical split with the past. His present struggle with dementia is his own, but the historical experiences he is describing are not merely unimportant, they are not even his.

The Malayan conflict has now largely been expunged from public memory. Never officially acknowledged as a war by the British government, it nevertheless involved 545,000 tons of explosives, the internment of 34,000 people, and the exfoliation of hundreds of acres of land. Hostilities in Malaysia continued for almost 20 years from 1948 to 1966. Until 1960, this was a war fought by conscripts on National Service. It is not surprising that having been involved in such a conflict should continue to loom large in someone's memory in a literal, rather than metaphorical, way.

In a later publication, Kitwood (1998) does in fact make *one* reference to a historical event triggering a distressed reaction in a person living with dementia. He outlines a role play exercise in which he took on the character of Richard, a man living in a residential home about whose life history very little is known. The participants are asked to note down clues about Richard's life story. Part of the mystery to be unfolded is Richard's single reference to 'Anzio', as he cowers under a table following a loud noise. Kitwood (1998,106) remarks that some participants 'even thought that Anzio was a person and had no inkling that it was the scene of a famous landing in World War II where there was heavy loss of life'. Given that Kitwood's own rendering of the 20th century is otherwise entirely without a war; this is something of a low punch.

The problem, as I am trying to re-frame it here, is that Kitwood would hold hard-pressed, underpaid care staff doing their best in a difficult situation responsible for the deterioration which takes place in people with dementia. Yet at no point does he place responsibility on wider social regimes, power structures, social inequalities or forms of discrimination that have affected people now living with dementia throughout the entirety of their pre-diagnosis lives. This seems to me to be not only morally wrong, but to miss the important point that very often the deterioration in question can better be understood as the reactivation of traumatic events from previous life, whether in everyday life, in social and national history, or at the interstices between the two. The citizenship and human rights literature which has begun to emerge since the 2010s (e.g. Bartlett and O'Connor 2010; Cahill 2022; and see Chapter 11 by Jenkins and Williamson) has made welcome inroads into re-framing dementia in its broader social contexts, but there is still a need in critical dementia studies for more attuned historical sensibilities.

Intersectionality and historical trauma

Time has moved on since Kitwood wrote his major work *Dementia Reconsidered* 25 years ago. This passage of time has also shifted on the parameters of our historical frame of reference by 25 years. We are no longer looking at the experience of

people whose 'reminiscence bump' years were between 1900 and 1925 or therea-
bouts, but from approximately 1925 to the 1970s. Only those who are now approaching their 100th birthday will have experienced World War II (WWII) as
adults. There are still plenty of people living with dementia today who remember
bombing raids and evacuation as children or teenagers, but their numbers will also
dwindle over the coming years.

It is easy to assume that because we have left behind that era of global conflict,
genocidal ideology and mass displacement, this means that a historical perspective will become unnecessary. Yet the post-WWII world has been characterised
by numerous postcolonial conflicts, the cold war, nuclear threat, famines, successive waves of forced migration and diasporas, an increase in natural disasters and
extreme weather conditions due to climate change, pandemic disease, increases in
online personal, sexual and financial abuse, among various other social ills. There
are also new cohorts of veterans and survivors reaching the at-risk years for onset
of dementia, from the Vietnam war to the Troubles in Northern Ireland and the
invasions of Afghanistan and Iran from disasters such as the collapse of the Twin
Towers, the Asian Tsunami and Hurricane Katrina to name only a few.

In all of these cases, large numbers of people underwent severely traumatic
experiences that are likely to be relived in the context of dementia. We know that
a significant proportion of survivors will go on to develop dementia. For example,
Brooks et al (2022) found that 80% of older African Americans reported having experienced trauma and Bhattarai et al (2019) found that black veterans in the United
States who had been diagnosed with conflict-related PTSD had almost double the
risk of developing dementia than those without such a diagnosis. We have never
done, and are still not doing anything like enough to prepare for this. There are, for
examples, huge implications here for staff education on trauma-informed practice,
and also – as other chapters in this text also point out – for acknowledging that
shared experiences of trauma are a way of connecting people with and without a
diagnosis of dementia as one community, not as 'us' and 'them'. People living with
dementia have, indeed, much to teach the world about survival.

Clearly, there are profound ethical dilemmas around such work. People who are
living with dementia may not choose to disclose troubling aspects of their life history at all, or they may do so inadvertently. Paying close attention to things someone
may be trying to convey and keeping any sensitive information confidential are obviously vital, but so are being prepared to do some research into local, social, national
and international history. This is clearly a tall order; however, merely by knowing
someone's age and where they have lived during their life it is possible to discover
much about the kind of events they may have experienced. To do this well takes time
and patience, and this is yet another reason why careworkers and other providers of
dementia services are not paid anywhere near enough for what they do.

Intersectionality is a term often used to represent multiple dimensions of difference affecting the same person synchronically (see an excellent discussion of
the term and its history by Lotherington in Chapter 6). That is to say a person can,
for example, be simultaneously disabled, black, queer and working class. Similarly, every person with a diagnosis of dementia will also have other dimensions of

intersectionality, including age, gender, sexuality, ethnicity and social class. Roes et al (2022) suggest that intersectionality is a concept that can help to avoid exclusion and discrimination for people with dementia. In this case, however, we also need to take into account that most of the person's formative experiences took place in times that were different (and in some cases, very different) from our own. For this reason, it seems to me that intersectionality, as the term is applied to people living with dementia, should also have a diachronic dimension; it should engage with how things have changed over time, recognising that these formative experiences may now become more salient once again, as a result of an increased reliance on remote and emotional memory to explain what is happening in the present day.

In the context of dementia, then, intersectionality only makes sense if we take a long view, and if we recognise that memories are not only held collectively within communities but also transmitted from generation to generation. In communities where there has been a history of lynch mobs, for example, an individual may hold this as a collective, embodied memory even though it never happened to them personally. Parental tension and hypervigilance can be handed down from parents to children in the form of intergenerational trauma. If an individual with this legacy also has a disability, these two dimensions of intersectionality interpenetrate to affect the way they experience their body; as, for example, an already historically threatened body that now cannot move quickly enough to escape. If the person in question also has dementia, he or she may be less able to understand that the original traumatic event is not happening again. The presence of uniformed white people in positions of authority is likely to be panic-inducing, regardless of whether their actual intentions are malignant or benign.

Our attention is repeatedly drawn to the number of people living with dementia; 850,000 in the UK alone we are told, 55 million globally. Yet far less consideration is given to the demographic implications of these numbers. Gender has finally been recognised as a factor in the experience of dementia, with two-thirds of those with a diagnosis being women. Logically, from a historical perspective, however, these women must include a significant number who were forced to give up children for adoption through homes for unmarried mothers, and the Magdalen Laundries. They must include former sex workers, women who had backstreet abortions, and women whose children died of diseases that we now barely know the names of – polio, diphtheria, pleurisy. We don't hear about this in mainstream life history work; instead we hear about women working as school dinner ladies and doing flower arranging. Intersectionality is a useful concept to the extent that it helps to remind us that people living with dementia are not homogenised by their diagnosis. But in order to understand the true heterogeneity of the population of people living with dementia, we need also to combine it with a well-developed historical consciousness.

Conclusion

As debate elsewhere in this book demonstrates, since Kitwood, there has been significant work on gender (Chapters 7 and 8), ethnicity (Chapter 9), citizenship (Chapter 10), human rights and posthumanism (Chapter 12), the fourth age, and precarity (see, for example, Chapter 10, by Grenier and Phillipson (2023), in the previous volume in this series *Critical Dementia Studies: An Introduction*). We have also seen the application of new bodies of social and critical theory; for example, perspectives drawn from the work of Bakhtin (Capstick and Chatwin 2016), Foucault (Knifton and Yates 2019) and Agamben (Burke 2019). There is clearly still, however, a significant theory-practice divide in dementia studies, and Kitwood's person-centred model seems extremely hard to shake, particularly in the practice field. In this chapter, I have tried to show why I believe this model to be not only incomplete, or unhelpful but also inimical to the interests both of people living with dementia and paid caregivers. I have suggested that people living with dementia have much to teach us about forgotten histories. I have also argued that the extent of historical trauma is under-recognised in people living with dementia, and that this has a great deal of impact on their lived experience in current day contexts of care and service provision. I suggest that rather than the malignant social psychology posited by Kitwood, it is the return of this historical trauma that explains much of the distressed behaviour of people living with dementia, particularly in long-term care, hospital environments or other forms of institution. Finally, I have suggested that we can only have a rounded awareness of intersectionality in the context of dementia if we bring a historical perspective to this project, as well as an awareness of dimensions of difference in the present day. By historicising dementia studies, not only do we become better able to communicate with people living with dementia, we also become more adept in using their testimony to challenge social amnesia.

References

Alwin, D. F. (2012) Integrating Varieties of Life Course Concepts. *The Journals of Gerontology: Series B*, 67B(2): 206–220. DOI: 10.1093/geronb/gbr146

Bartlett, R. & O'Connor, D. (2010) *Broadening the Dementia Debate*. Cambridge: Policy Press.

Bhattarai, J. J., Oehlert, M. E., Multon, K. D. & Sumerall, S. W. (2019) Dementia and Cognitive Impairment among U.S. Veterans with a History of MDD or PTSD: A Retrospective Cohort Study based on Sex and Race. *Journal of Aging and Health*, 31(8): 1398–1422. DOI: 10.1177/0898264318781131

Brooks, J. R., Taylor, R. J. & Chatteers, L. M. (2022) The Impact of Traumatic Events on Mental Health among Older African American and Black Caribbean Adults. *Journal of Aging and Health*, 34(3): 390–400. DOI: 10.1177/08982643221086336

Brown, M. & Clegg, D. (Eds.) (2007) *Ancient Mysteries*. London: The Trebus Publishing.

Bryce, C., Capstick, A., Cinamon, G., Clegg, D., Davis, P. E. H., Fairchild, G., Greenberger, D., Hawley, E., & Hesketh, S. (2010) *Tell Mrs Mill Her Husband Is Still Dead*. London: The Trebus Publishing.

Burke, L. (2019) Dementia and the Paradigm of the Camp: Thinking beyond Giorgio Agamben's Concept of 'Bare Life. *Journal of Bioethical Inquiry*, 16(2):195–205.

Cahill, S. (2022) New Analytical Tools and Frameworks to Understand Dementia: What can a Human Rights Lens Offer. *Ageing and Society*, 42, 1489–1498.

Capstick, A. & Chatwin, J. (2016) The Carnival is Not Over: Cultural Resistance in Dementia Care Environments. *Pragmatics and Society*, 7(2): 169–195.

Capstick, A. & Clegg, D. (2013) Behind the Stiff Upper Lip: War Narratives of Older Men with Dementia. *Journal of War and Culture Studies*, 6(3): 239–254.

Capstick, A. & Ludwin, K. (2015) Place Memory and Dementia: Findings from Participatory Film-making in Long-term Care. *Health and Place*, 34: 157–163.

Cheston, R. (1996) Stories and Metaphors: Talking about the Past in a Psychotherapy Group for People with Dementia. *Ageing and Society*, 16: 579–602.

Gove, D., Beatty, A., Capstick, A., Ettenes, P., Georges, J., Gzil, F., Harper, P., Rohra, H., Sandberg, L., Scerri, A., Scerri, C., Schumacher-Dimech, A. & Westerlund, K. (2022). *Sex, Gender and Sexuality in the Context of Dementia: A Discussion Paper*. Luxembourg: Alzheimer Europe.

Grenier, A. & Phillipson, C. (2023) Precarity and Dementia. In Ward, R. and Sandberg, L. (Eds.) *Critical Dementia Studies: An Introduction*. London: Routledge.

Jacoby, R (1996) *Social Amnesia: A Critique of Contemporary Psychology*. London: Transaction.

Kitwood, T. (1990) Understanding Senile Dementia: A Psychobiographical Approach. *Free Associations*, 19: 60–76.

Kitwood, T. (1997) *Dementia Reconsidered: The Person Comes First*. Buckingham: Open University Press.

Kitwood, T. (1998) Life History and Its Vestiges. In Schweitzer P (Ed.) *Reminiscence in Dementia Care*. London: Age Concern: 103–107.

Knifton, C. & Yates, S. (2019) A 'History of Problematizations' for Dementia Education: A Foucauldian Approach to Understanding the Framing of Dementia. *Journal of Research in Nursing*, 24(3–4): 212–230. DOI: 10.1177/1744987119831737

Kruger-Fürhoff, I. M., Schmidt, N. and Vice, S. (2021) *The Politics of Dementia: Forgetting and Remembering the Violent Past in Literature, Film and Graphic Narratives*. Berlin: De Gruyter.

Roes, M., Laporte Uribe, F., Peters-Nehrenheim, V., Smits, C., Lohannessen, A., Charlesworth, G. M., Parveen, S., Muller, N., Hedd Jones, C., Thyrian, J. R., Monsees, J & Tezcan, H. (2022) Intersectionality and Its Relevance for Research in Dementia Care of People with a Migration Background. *Zeitschrift für Gerontologie + Geriatrie*, 55(4). DOI: 10.1007/s00391-022-02058

Saad G. (2019) *An Introduction to Trauma in Early Childhood*. Georgetown: University of Georgetown. https://gucchd.georgetown.edu/projects/docs/Introduction%20to%20Trauma%20in%20EC%20PPT.pdf

Smail, D. (1993) *The Origins of Unhappiness: A New Understanding of Personal Distress*. London: HarperCollins.

Thomsen, D. K and Berntsen, D (2008) The Cultural Life Script and Life Story Chapters Contribute to the Reminiscence Bump. *Memory*, 16 (4): 420–435.

UK Life Story Network www.lifestorynetwork.org.uk

Part II
Discourses

3   Language about people with dementia

*Clare Mason, Michael Andrews, Ronald Ferguson
(aka Ronald Amanze), Jacqui Bingham, Allison
Batchelor, Gerald King, Teresa Davies (aka Dory),
Julie Hayden, and Wendy Mitchell*

Introduction

Language can influence how we 'think and behave' and can indicate that a person lacks ability (Wilson et al., 2021). The way we talk to and about people with dementia has been described as contributing to the 'social death' of those with a diagnosis (George 2010). Many argue that stigma related to dementia plays a large part in how we as the public, view and communicate with those with a diagnosis (Swaffer 2014). (For a discussion of language used about dementia, and people living with dementia, in an international context, see Chapter 4, by Koncul and colleagues). The Oxford English Dictionary describes stigma as 'a mark of disgrace associated with a particular circumstance, quality, or person'. However, stigma means many different things to different people. For the authors, the word stigma is felt to conjure up an image of society keeping us at arm's length because they are unsure and ignorant of the facts; to be ashamed of, or a fear of being labelled. We also feel it is a form of discrimination. It is felt to be unintentional by the person doing it, usually due to a lack of understanding of dementia.

When looking at stigma against dementia, Alzheimer's Society Canada provides a good description of it; stigma against dementia encompasses any negative attitude or discriminatory behaviour against people living with dementia. Stigma also involves negative attitudes or discrimination against someone based on a distinguishing characteristic such as a mental illness, as unfair thoughts and views of a person who is different from yourself. These are set on unfounded, inaccurate ideas which lead on to treating the stigmatised person or people in a way which can cause long-term trauma and can influence the way others see people who are grouped in a similar way according to race, disability, creed or social standing. It is also felt that stigma is when other people presume, they know what it is like to have dementia and they 'believe they know what I need and what I want'.

The way people speak to, and about people living with dementia can, as author Wendy Mitchell (2018a) has noted, 'make or break' a person. Philly Hare, of *Innovations in Dementia* (n.d.) has highlighted that negative language used in reference to people with dementia can instil fear in younger people about approaching old age, sensationalising the illness, and that the most offensive words used are typically attached to the person rather than the condition itself (Hare 2014).

DOI: 10.4324/9781003290353-6

There is a growing movement of people living with dementia who actively speak out about dementia and the language used towards them. Those able to speak out often vocalise how they are doing their best to live well with dementia and how the negative language used around dementia is undoing much of this work.

This chapter is co-authored by people living with dementia who are members of DEEP (Dementia Engagement and Empowerment Project). It describes some of the language used towards us and the impact it has had. The authors of this chapter are members of the University of Bradford, Centre for Applied Dementia Studies, Experts by Experience Group, and the Pathways young onset dementia support group. Language is a topic which is frequently discussed during both group meetings and something we all feel strongly about as an area for concern. Clare Mason, a dementia care trainer, and Experts by Experience lead at the University of Bradford, worked with the Experts by Experience to collate their views and experiences of language in relation to dementia for this chapter. To collect the information for this chapter, we met on Zoom, an online conferencing platform, due to the geographical spread of members, to discuss the topic. We also contributed to the chapter by email. Clare Mason collated each section and we then exchanged amendments, additions and corrections by email. (It is worth reading this chapter alongside Chapter 12, by the Scottish Alumni Group, regarding their experiences of dementia advocacy.)

Also included are some extracts from a Pathways young onset dementia support group online forum, demarcated in this chapter within textboxes. These are comments posted by people with dementia, current and former family carers and paid carers and we believe that they give a wider viewpoint on the use of language in relation to dementia. An article posted on the Pathways young onset dementia Facebook page titled 'How not to talk about dementia' had 380 views and 4 shares, demonstrating the strength of feeling and level of interest in this topic. In a recent Twitter debate, many people posted about how the media uses language that describes them as being a burden to their families and to society (Talbot et al., 2020).

Historical terminology

Looking back over the last 30 years at the way people have referred to and communicated with people living with dementia, much of the terminology has, thankfully, changed. However, some of this language has remained. There are many historical terms which have been used to describe people living with dementia. We consider many of these to be hurtful and condescending, but they were used, nonetheless. Such terms include 'away with the fairies', 'ready for the loony bin', 'pleasantly puddled' and 'tapped in the head'. People were afraid of 'being put away', which is a term often heard by some of us to describe those who might be sent to live in an institution. The name dementia derives from the Latin word 'demens' and is described as a person who is 'out of their mind'. The phrase 'out of one's mind' is still used today. We have heard people say, 'He's going on a (dementia) journey' or that a person with dementia is an 'empty shell'. One phrase that we have heard used by a health professional is 'Dementia is like an onion, with the layers taken away'. Other terms that we have experienced are that the person is 'fading away' or 'disappearing' or going 'dotty'. In our experience, people say these things jokingly, like 'He's a couple of pennies short' or 'has a few 'slates' missing', but it is still hurtful.

There are also terms that we have heard both in dementia training sessions, from care staff and in our own personal experience, over the last 20 years or so, to be used to describe people such as those living in care homes. People would be described as a bed number in a hospital dementia ward or a room number in a care setting. These terms are believed to dehumanise people and are part of what Tom Kitwood (1997) described as the old culture care, where people had things done to them rather than with them as a collaborative effort (Capstick considers Kitwood's critique in Chapter 2). This old culture of care was focussed on disability, rather than ability, stripping people of their identity and sense of self.

Historically, people who were given a diagnosis of 'senile dementia', another derogatory term, were placed in institutions and asylums. There were institutions or asylums in most local areas, where people simply 'disappeared' to (Fletcher discusses the historic use of 'senile dementia' in Chapter 1). Much of the language used towards and about people with dementia during this time was a form of labelling, rarely using a person's name or using a person-centred approach which sees the person first and the dementia second. One such setting in Bradford closed as recently as 2003. Some of us who live locally remember this as a place to be feared, where people were referred to as 'inmates', like those who lived in prisons and had committed crimes. The word 'dementia' was rarely used in reference to these people and their disappearances, due to the fear and horror felt by those who realised what had taken place and that it might also one day happen to them.

People with dementia were often described as having a 'second childhood'. We still hear this spoken of today. It is used when referring to someone who has impaired short-term memory and perpetuates the belief that they are younger than they are, perhaps still a child or a teenager. It is also used to describe people who need care like that of a child, such as support to use the toilet, eat, dress or bathe. It gives little value to the fact that people with dementia have had lives and learned how to do these things, but due to cognitive impairment and other disabilities are no longer able to.

Today, we are often described as having 'mental health issues' and caution is advised when interacting with us as we may become aggressive due to cognitive impairment. DEEP member Michael said:

> I don't like the term "mental health issues". It can mean a number of things, if someone has killed someone and goes to court, they use this to get a lesser sentence.

At a recent debate, which took place at a Scottish dementia conference, about changing the word 'dementia', Gerry, who lives with young onset dementia and was at the conference, said:

> 'I don't mind the word "dementia", it's like the word "cancer", it just describes an illness'.

Historically, this was not a common view. Support groups for people with dementia were given other, softer titles and dementia cafes were termed 'well-being cafes' or 'memory cafes' to prevent people being put off by the use of the word 'dementia'. People were referred to as having 'memory problems' and a dementia support worker would contact potential 'clients' by explaining their work as working with people with memory problems, even though it is well known that memory loss or memory problems are not the only symptoms of dementia.

In the 1990s, the term 'person with dementia' started to be used in texts books and other publications, rather than 'dementia sufferer' (discussed further below) or 'patient' outside of a medical context. Julie Hayden, who is a former nurse and social worker, now living with dementia, adds:

> 'Simply calling us 'people' would be nice – but when we're referred to as patients, that is felt by some to be infuriating. Unless I'm in a doctor's surgery or a hospital, I'm a person, not a patient'.

However, this view is not shared by all. Some of us feel that the use of the term 'patient' either in hospital or in a GP (General Practitioner) surgery, is more acceptable as it is used to describe all who use those services, not just people with a dementia diagnosis.

Interpersonal communication

Some of us feel that once the word 'dementia' is used or directed at us, we become invisible. The word in itself is inoffensive, but it is what happens once the word is used that can be upsetting. For instance, in our experience, once a person receives a diagnosis, professionals often speak to the carer or family member, rather than the person with the diagnosis. Alison Batchellor of Northern Ireland said:

> 'My husband is really, really supportive but in one meeting, I actually had to stop it as the whole focus was on him, and the meeting was supposed to be about me'.

Many of us have had similar experiences. We believe that more education is needed to support those who attempt to communicate with a person with dementia. There appears to be a lack of knowledge on how to speak with and to a person living with dementia and people need education on 'how to speak *to us* rather than going through somebody else to speak *about us*'. On this topic, Michael and Julie said respectively:

> 'People don't know what they don't know'.
> 'It is our job as educators to help others understand why language is so important and the impact it can have on those on the receiving end of it'.

We believe that it would be far better if people just asked, rather than assumed. Many of us are involved in other meetings and activities where topics such as 'assumptions' are discussed. We feel that making assumptions about a person with dementia's abilities, disabilities, wants, needs and preferences can be dangerous or. at least, disrespectful. The danger is that an assumption is made that a person wants a certain thing at a certain time, yet they are not consulted or asked. They may respond in the only way they are able, maybe shouting or pushing a person away. They are then labelled as aggressive or as having challenging behaviour. This could be avoided by use of appropriate language and not making assumptions and holding pre-conceived ideas. In another context, Jacqui Bingham who lives in Stockport, has experienced difficulties with the way people speak to her at Church:

> 'People will often say to my friend, even though we're side by side "How's Jacqui?" and will then turn to me and speak to me in a really condescending voice. It's not just about language, but the way a person speaks, their tone of voice, as well as the words they use'.

At times, it is very hard not to laugh when people speak in this manner, but some of us, particularly when we are experiencing a bad day, can be offended by it and that can put us off attending Church or other community groups or events.

The way people speak to us, either using 'inappropriate language' or a condescending tone of voice or demeanour, not only has an impact on us as the people with dementia who are being spoken to or about. Our friends and family are also affected and can often lose confidence in going out with us. They are also reluctant to join us in activities or outings, maybe going to the pub or a restaurant or other public places. This can lead to feelings of isolation, resentment and abandonment, a feeling of being different and not accepted by our circle of friends or our wider communities and even worse, our families.

Institutional language

Historically, institutions such as care homes and hospitals have used negative language in documents such as care plans, reports and correspondence. A care home, where one author previously worked, had lists of residents who needed assistance with eating at mealtimes displayed on the dining room wall with the heading 'feeders', another on the toilet wall was labelled 'doubles' for those people who needed two members of staff to assist them to use the bathroom, or 'pads' for those who wore incontinence pads. This negativity implies that people are seen as objects and things are done to them rather than with them. It also creates an image of dependence and disability. Similarly, we have found that many organisations use 'interventions' and 'tools', all far from human terms, implying that these are used 'on' people with dementia and are far from collaborative. Social media platforms such as Twitter and Facebook are awash with medics, researchers and clinicians posting about their latest 'toolkit' or 'intervention' for people with dementia, again reinforcing the 'being done to' element of old culture care.

In our experience, a common term used in institutional settings is 'non-compliance'. This is used when a person refuses to do what is expected or asked of them by a professional. Describing this, Julie Hayden explains:

'If I change my mind about doing something or show reluctance, or simply just can't be bothered to do something at the time a professional ask or suggests it, I'm labelled as "non-compliant". It makes my blood boil, I have a right to change my mind and a right to make unwise decisions, or at very least, make a decision about my own care'.

We believe that the biggest change in institutional language needs to come from the medical world. We have found the diagnosis process to be full of negative language because it follows the medical model – 'failed', 'reduced', 'can't', 'nothing I can do'. If only medical professionals balanced their clinical expertise with the social model of focussing on what the person can still do, we would receive a diagnosis that leaves us with a feeling of a life still to be lived instead of a future of despair, simply by changing the language used. It would cost them nothing to change. Julie Hayden said:

'I'm so ashamed of my profession, I was a social worker in older people's services and the language they use and the attitudes I get from social services is truly awful. There's a big problem by the fact I'm on my own and I'm always on my own with them so they think it's okay to use this derogatory language that continues to offend and belittle me'.

When an ambulance was called for Teresa Davies who lives with young onset dementia, one ambulance crew member said to their colleague: 'We have a dementia'. Teresa described this as having a very negative impact on her at the time.

The concept of citizenship in relation to dementia contends that people with dementia have a right to participate in society on their own terms, and that their human rights should be upheld. However, language such as 'non-compliance' implies that people with dementia should be grateful for any help offered or given, rather than support being a right or entitlement.

For us, the use of language by professionals is vitally important as this can affect the level of trust a person has with individual professionals and, in turn, organisations. It can also affect whether a person takes up a service or not or engages in a support group or activity. Ronald, who lives in Luton and has young onset dementia, explains that professionals often ask him about the 'support' he is receiving:

> 'I'm not looking for support, I'm looking for meaningful things to do, to collaborate and share my ideas. One of the worst types of language I experience is the silent language. Where you can hear the things, they don't' say, you can see it in their eyes. They're looking at you and silently saying that you're one of the needy people who needs to be cared for. Silent language, attitude, tone you can see it in their eyes. They're thinking you're just one of the needy people'.
>
> They're thinking of you as one of the needy people or unruly people. When you try to assert yourself, or speak up about what you feel, you can run the risk of being told that you're being aggressive or angry or get defined as being a problem'.

We hold a common belief that language used by professionals can be damaging and demeaning. Some people put the onus on the person with dementia by making us feel like *we* are the problem and that this makes situations very complicated. Jacqui shared her experience:

> 'Because of the Covid, I've had to have some discussions on the phone. One lady wanted to tell me about a colonoscopy. She went through three pages of telling me how they do it. Even though I told her I didn't want it. I didn't get unruly, I just said "No". "No, I don't want it". She spoke to me in a really sarcastic tone, and I nearly put the phone down. It's not the first time this has happened, I think professionals are taught how to speak with someone who has dementia; they speak to you and use language that makes me feel like a little girl'.

The use of language in relation to people with dementia can be far worse when a person is on their own and doesn't have another person to speak on their behalf. We have experienced attitudes change when professionals learn that you are on your own. There seems to be no regard for the fact that a person may have once been a professional themselves, lived an independent life, raised a family or had a position in their local community. It feels like professionals often forget the person they are 'dealing' with is a person in their own right, with thoughts, feelings and emotions.

The way language is used by organisations such as care providers, councils and benefits agencies can also come across as discriminatory. In some instances, we can be reluctant to apply for financial benefits due to the terms used in application forms. In particular, the example below of the terms used to apply for a reduction in council tax causes a great deal of controversy and anger.

To apply for council tax disregard, to enable a person to receive a reduction in council tax, we must first be confirmed as having 'severe mental impairment' by a doctor. Some of us have refused to apply for it due to this terminology and labelling. Michael Andrews, originally from Northern Ireland, now living in Bradford who has posterior cortical atrophy dementia, wrote on the Pathways support group online forum:

> 'I hate that term, severely mentally impaired, and then you fill in the forms and then your doctor has to confirm it, and some doctors will say you have dementia but you're not severely mentally impaired, so then the council won't let you have the reduction. It used to be if you had a diagnosis you were entitled to it, but then the government changed the name, some people refused to apply for it because of the way it was worded and some doctors would not sign the forms, so it is saving the government and councils money, but I do agree it has to change, this is a way the council can discriminate on someone trying to claim benefits, by using the way they call it. They don't recognise the word dementia and you have to fill forms out to say that you are severely mentally impaired. Then some fill out the forms to find that their doctor won't confirm it, then they get refused the benefit and then if you are getting the benefit, you have to go through the forms each year, and they only give you so many days to reply or you lose your benefit. Each year it's getting harder and harder'.

When completing an application for council tax disregard, the language used in the form, which focusses on disability rather than abilities, weaknesses rather than strengths, and dependence rather than independence, can make people feel like a complete failure and totally worthless.

Suffering and sufferer

Over recent years, one term which has inspired much debate is 'suffering' and, relatedly, 'sufferer' (Bös & Schneider 2022). In her daily blog entitled *Which me am I today?* best-selling author, Wendy Mitchell, who lives with dementia, writes that 'fighting' incurable cancer and other illnesses is often spoken about, but that those with these illnesses want to show the positive side of their illnesses, just like people with dementia'. She asks: 'So why is 'suffering' acceptable for people with dementia but not for other illnesses?' (Mitchell 2018b). Language can define a person, so the psychological effect of words should never be underestimated. Most editors or journalists get it when told, but headlines are often thought of at the last minute by another journalist who has not had those conversations. This leads to headlines such as 'dementia sufferer' being used. When we read this, it can feel like a betrayal of all the trust put in the journalist.

We all have different perspectives of what the word 'suffering' means. Most of us do not feel we suffer. Having good days and bad days comes with any illness or disability. It is not unique to dementia. Gerry wrote:

> 'I find the word "dementia sufferer" very offensive, I think people need to be really careful. It's really quite offensive and I'd far rather be referred to as having dementia. My kids call me some horrible words and I see that as just fun, being called a sufferer is awful'.

Allison Batchellor, who lives with young onset dementia in Northern Ireland, wrote:

> 'If someone calls me a "dementia sufferer", I quickly correct them, explaining that dementia is a condition I have, it's not something I suffer with or from. Most people don't mean it, but I do correct them'.

As far back as 1992, Tom Kitwood, the founder of Bradford Dementia Group and a pioneer of person-centred dementia care, and Kathleen Bredin (Kitwood & Bredin 1992) wrote that 'Dementia involves a lot of suffering for both the person who is affected and for others who are close'. However, they went on to say that not all the suffering is related solely to brain damage and the impact it has, but that some of the suffering came about because it was not known, then, how to best care for a person with dementia.

People can suffer with dementia because of the way other people treat them and because of how they are represented. For instance, the term 'sufferer' is widely used, in books, magazines and in the media, as well as in esteemed journals such as the *British Medical Journal*. As recently as May 2022, the National Health Service in Oxfordshire published a document online with the words 'dementia sufferer's daughter' in the heading (NHS 2022). The article goes on to describe how Penny Marsh's mother suffered with dementia for four years. Bös and Schneider (2022) have described the use of terms such as 'sufferer' as having an impact on society, positioning people with dementia as passive victims. We believe that those referring to people with dementia, in particular, researchers, have a responsibility to readjust their language to minimise its impact.

The word 'suffering' is often used by those without a diagnosis of dementia. Like people living with other disabilities, we can lack the confidence to correct people, and can instead withdraw into ourselves, disengaging from conversations.

This can result in us being viewed as 'awkward' or 'miserable' when it can actually be a form of self-preservation and a protective mechanism against hurtful comments and negative interactions. At a recent dementia conference in Wales, a person with dementia, who was a key speaker, used the phrase 'people suffering from dementia' and we heard a loud boo and light-hearted jeering from the audience, its members being mostly those with a diagnosis and those either caring for them or with a particular interest in it. However, Julie Hayden suggests that we should not make others feel guilty of using such terms:

'After all, you don't know what you don't know. Making people fearful of saying the wrong thing, putting them off speaking with us, only adds to the stigma and isolation faced by many of us on a daily basis. The term 'sufferer' has become quite a contentious issue and just feeds back into the stigma. People who are really struggling, really having severe symptoms, and their relatives will often say they are suffering. What they're really saying is they're seeing me as not suffering and that I'm okay – it's a very tricky area. I think we've got to be as understanding as we can about any alternatives. We need to say, look, I'm living as well as I can with it. I do struggle, but for the most part I'm concentrating on living as well as I can with it. suffering can be used appropriately when self-referencing by a person according to how they feel about their condition. However, it's inappropriate to extrapolate that across to all people that live with dementia'.

Living well

As mentioned, over recent years, another term which has been commonly used when talking about people living with dementia is 'living well'. Some have considered this to be a more positive way of framing dementia and it has become widely used in organisations such as the Alzheimer's Society, Dementia UK and other organisations working to support people with dementia and their families. Some believe it is possible to live well with dementia by keeping socially and physically active, keeping connected to social groups and communities and having meaningful things to do. Living well is referred to throughout the Dementia Guide, a book produced for people living with dementia by the NHS and Alzheimer's Society (2013). In many ways, using the term 'living well' with dementia can give a person hope that it is possible to live well. However, for some of us this feels contradictory to the difficulties we are experiencing or the experiences of some family members when witnessing the perceived struggles of their relatives.

Many people who understand dementia or those who have taken time to find out about it have typically use the phrase 'living with dementia' rather than 'suffering'. We believe that those who do not like the term 'living with dementia' may be seeking attention or sympathy and want people to feel sorry for them. This mostly relates to those who find themselves in a position of caring for a person with a diagnosis. In the online young onset dementia forum Pathways, one family carer wrote:

> 'You can't battle dementia, once it's got you that's it. You can try and live well with it for as long as you can but ultimately, it's a death sentence as there is no cure. People who have dementia are not always aware they are a sufferer; I think the sufferer is the carer as they know exactly what's in store for the person they look after. The key word here is "thankfully". You just have to get on with life and do the very best you can to get as much as possible from it while you have the chance'.

Here, using the term 'sufferer' demonstrates the burden they feel they are carrying. Hence, the word 'suffering' can be a key part of a family carers' identity and speaks to how the family carer views the person they are caring for and their situation, and possibly how it is impacting on their life and their family life, and how it prevents them living the life they once lived. When speaking at a Welsh dementia conference about her own experience, Glenda, who lives with dementia said:

> 'When you get a diagnosis of dementia, your whole family gets a diagnosis'.

Glenda's statement was met with huge cheers from the audience and echoes of agreement. Hence, it is important to acknowledge that carers and family members can feel that they are unable to 'live well' themselves.

Some of us feel that we do not live well with dementia, and some of us feel we live as well with dementia as one can. We believe that, to live well with dementia, you have to make changes to your life. You have to come up with strategies such as using technology and gadgets to live as well as you can, in the best way you can. As time and dementia progress, adjustments have to be made and strategies tweaked. However, it is important that the gadgets and technology are used to enhance independence rather than take over our remaining abilities. Gadgets and technology are used by many of us, but they cannot help with language or speech, and this is frustrating for some.

Dementia friendly, says who?

Several years ago, the Alzheimer's Society in the UK began the 'Dementia Friends' (n.d.) initiative to create greater awareness and respect for the needs of people with dementia within communities and the businesses and organisations that serve them. This was part of the Society's five-year plan and became part of the Prime Minister's Challenge 2012 (DoH 2012). The term 'dementia friendly' was introduced, with organisations being given the opportunity to work towards becoming 'dementia friendly'. This was originally envisaged as organisations and businesses being given this status if they had taken the time to learn about dementia, so that they could create environments where people with dementia are understood, respected and supported. Organisations would also make a pledge as to how they were going to support people with dementia within their premises or when using their services. As becoming a dementia friendly organisation was considered an ongoing process, organisations received a sticker carrying the Dementia Friends logo for their shop window. They could use this to announce they were 'working towards' being dementia friendly once they had registered with the process.

The term 'friendly' in itself is considered interesting by the authors, 'it was thought by many of those working in the field of dementia at the time and is still a widespread belief of many, that if places are adapted and made easier, so 'friendly' for people with dementia, they would be easier for all, especially those with a disability, such as visual impairment or a physical disability. Although initially, this referred to the physical environment, it now appears to refer to approach and attitude of those without dementia, towards those who are diagnosed with it.

Over recent years, this well-intentioned campaign has lost favour with many dementia activists (Rahman & Swaffer 2018). Adopted by many, but unregulated, businesses have displayed dementia friendly stickers for many years after attending only one awareness session and having undergone many subsequent changes of staff. Health authorities have replaced dementia training workshops for frontline staff with Dementia Friends creation opportunities which are led by people who have only attended a one-day introduction to the method of their delivery.

Some of these Dementia Friends Champions are themselves living with a diagnosis and so can provide greater insight into the true meaning of dementia, but most are not. It is vital that health and social care professionals are given dementia training and not merely awareness presentations as a cheap alternative, as they will never be fit for purpose. They are inadequately detailed and can be focused on our disabilities rather than on our abilities if we are given a little assistance. It ceases to hold real meaning if a badge is awarded to an organisation and remains in situ for eternity without review of the quality-of-service delivery. The guiding light of how we can most effectively be enabled to remain as independent as possible lays with us. Accessing dementia friendly assistance means repeatedly disclosing our diagnosis, and many of our requirements coincide with those living with other conditions the best approach is through insightful environmental design which combats the issue of being fit for purpose for all, not just those living with dementia.

Does it make any difference?

Over the last 25 years, more universities have begun teaching dementia studies, including the University of Bradford, the University of Worcester, the University of Stirling, and others. The language used in relation to people living with dementia is often covered in teaching and learning material. We feel that this makes a difference to care practice, not only for those delivering and receiving the training but also for those living with dementia.

We believe that if the reason why appropriate use of language is important is explained to students, this is usually better understood. If there is input either directly or indirectly from a person with lived experience of dementia, this information is better received than if it is just given by a tutor. For example, in a University of Bradford dementia course, language used in relation to dementia is covered in detail and the DEEP (n.d.) 'Dementia Words Matter' guide, written by people living with dementia, is used as a resource for students, who are usually from care, nursing or hospice professions. Exercises where students are asked to think about situations where they themselves have experienced derogatory language and made to not feel like a person are explored, and the impact on their own behaviour and relationships is reflected upon. This is then discussed in relation to people living with dementia, where students are asked, if a person with dementia was in the same situation and made to not feel like a person by the treatment, language, or attitudes of another human being, would they respond and react any differently? Videos, case studies and direct examples of people living with dementia are used in this teaching, and course feedback often confirms that this has been more helpful than if it was a written text or presentation without the voice of a person with lived experience.

The negative impact of some of the words used when talking with a person living with dementia can be catastrophic, resulting in a lack of confidence, low self-esteem, increased anxiety and a reluctance or even refusal to attempt to enter into further engagement. Those without a dementia diagnosis have sometimes said to us that they are fearful of communicating with people with dementia for fear of saying the wrong thing. To this end, it is important that we who work within the field of dementia and those who live with a diagnosis educate people but do not alienate them, preventing them from interacting or even being in the same space as a person with dementia.

References

Alzheimer's Society. (2013). *The Dementia Guide: Living Well after Diagnosis*. https://www.alzheimers.org.uk/sites/default/files/2018-07/AS_NEW_The%20dementia%20guide_update%203_WEB.pdf

Bös, B., & Schneider, C. (2022). Dementia sufferer and person living with a diagnosis of dementia: Naming practices in academia. *Age, Culture, Humanities: An Interdisciplinary Journal*, doi: 10.7146/ageculturehumanities.v6i.133272.

DEEP. (n.d.). *Dementia Words Matter*. https://www.dementiaaction.org.uk/dementiawords

Dementia Friends. (n.d.). https://www.dementiafriends.org.uk/

DoH. (2012). Prime Minister's challenge on dementia: Delivering major improvements in dementia care and research by 2015. *Department of Health*. https://www.gov.uk/government/publications/prime-ministers-challenge-on-dementia

George, D. R. (2010). Overcoming the social death of dementia through language. *The Lancet*, 376(9741), 586–587.

Hare, P. (2014). Time bombs and tsunamis: the impact of negative language and images on people with dementia. *24th Alzheimer Europe Conference: Dignity and Autonomy in Dementia*. https://www.youtube.com/watch?v=1Qk3-gonW-U&ab_channel=AlzheimerEurope

Innovations in Dementia. (n.d.). http://www.innovationsindementia.org.uk/

Kitwood, T. (1997). *Dementia Reconsidered: The Person Comes First.* Buckingham: Open University Press.

Kitwood, T., & Bredin, K. (1992). *Person to Person: A Guide to the Care of Those with Failing Mental Powers.* Loughton: Gale Centre Publications.

Mitchell, W. (2018a). Somebody I used to know. *Hay Festival.* https://www.hayfestival.com/wales/blog.aspx?post=316

Mitchell, W. (2018b). To 'Suffer' or not to 'Suffer', that is the question…… *Which Me Am I Today?* https://whichmeamitoday.wordpress.com/2018/03/08/to-suffer-or-not-to-suffer-that-is-the-question/

NHS. (2022). *Dementia Sufferer's Daughter Calls for Research Volunteers.* Oxford Health NHS Foundation Trust. https://www.oxfordhealth.nhs.uk/news/dementia-sufferers-daughter-calls-for-research-volunteers/

Rahman, S., & Swaffer, K. (2018). Assets-based approaches and dementia-friendly communities. *Dementia*, 17(2), 131–137.

Swaffer, K. (2014). Dementia: Stigma, language, and dementia friendly. *Dementia*, 13(6), 709–716.

Talbot, C. V., O'Dwyer, S. T., Clare, L., Heaton, J., & Anderson, J. (2020). How people with dementia use twitter: A qualitative analysis. *Computers in Human Behavior*, 102, 112–119.

Wilson, C. B., Hinson, J., Wilson, J. L., Power, S., Hinson, D., & Petriwskyj, A. (2021). Theatre production: A positive metaphor for dementia care-giving. *Ageing & Society*, doi: 10.1017/S0144686X21000428

4 A semiotic analysis of meanings of dementia around the world

Ana Koncul, Elizabeth George Onyedikachi, and Ruth Bartlett

Introduction

This chapter represents an endeavour to develop a critical history of language in dementia studies. To contribute to such an effort, we open the discussion about language and consider how dementia is described in languages other than English, which has been the main focus of scholarly work in the field (for a recent example of discussion on the impact of terms in popular use in English, see Chapter 3, by Mason and colleagues). Namely, we look at French, Italian, Chinese, Norwegian, Swahili, Urdu, Russian and other Slavic languages to understand the meanings of dementia worldwide. These languages have been selected either because they are most widely spoken in the world (see Figure 4.1), due to their relevance for the way dementia is perceived in different cultures, and/or because there is a native speaker on the author team.

In addition to being one of the most widely spoken, French is also one of the most influential languages regarding dementia: while the word 'dementia' itself has

Figure 4.1 QR Code of Language Family Tree (Young & Sundberg, 2015)

DOI: 10.4324/9781003290353-7

roots in Latin, its use worldwide comes from French. Furthermore, all varieties of Chinese belong to a family of more than 400 languages. It is estimated that 16% of the world population speaks a variety of Chinese as their first language. Most of the 315 million Slavic speakers worldwide are concentrated in 13 Slavic countries in East, Southeast and Central Europe, as well as in Central and North Asia, making it one of the world's largest language groups. Russian is the most widely spoken Slavic language (see Table 4.1); hence, the main focus will be on the construction of the perception of dementia by means of the Russian language. Africa accounts for a third of the languages spoken around the world, with Swahili standing as one of the most widely used on the continent. Similarly, with millions of native speakers and more than 170 million people using Urdu as their second language – most of them coming from Pakistan, India and Nepal – it is one of the most widely spoken languages in the world. Together with Danish, Faroese, Icelandic and Swedish, Norwegian belongs to a family of North Germanic or Nordic languages, spoken by 20 million people around the world. Norwegian is one of the smallest languages we focus on in this chapter. Yet we do so because of the distinct approach to health and welfare exemplified in the so-called Nordic model, characteristic of publicly financed comprehensive healthcare systems, support for research and policy development for the prevention and treatment of dementia, to name a few. This chapter briefly reflects on several other cultures and societies in order to extend the debates about dis/abling language. It also traces the history of dementia further back than other works in this collection. This is to show how the language of dementia has changed and is changing due to cultural influences and shifts in professional thinking in the countries/continents where these languages are spoken.

We open the discussion by briefly defining two terms that are used throughout the chapter, namely semiotics and language. Next, we outline the importance of language to thinking and practice. Here we remind readers of the powerful role language can play in stigmatising people who live with dementia. The chapter further charts how the term dementia has been defined and how its meanings are interpreted in each of the selected languages. Our findings represent a snapshot of vocabulary used at the time of writing and show that most languages have derogatory terms for dementia. By looking at documents such as the Norwegian Dementia Plan 2025 (Demensplan 2025, 2020), we demonstrate how initially favoured replacement words are often themselves superseded in various languages and cultures.

Defining language and semiotics

Semiotics is a philosophical approach, theory, and methodology that seeks to identify and interpret meaning by analysing signs, words, images, texts and systems of signification such as language. This chapter employs semiotic analysis to identify and interpret how meanings are constructed, assigned to dementia, and communicated. We use semiotics to understand the meaning of dementia in selected languages by looking at the vocabulary related to it and the various connotations the words bear. We look at the etymology, synonyms, jargon, symbolism, texts as well as the potential future related to the official vocabulary.

Table 4.1 Meaning of dementia in various languages[2]

Language	Language family	Number of speakers	Noun	Translation (English)	Synonyms in original language	Synonyms (translated to English)
French	Romance	275 million	la démence	dementia	aberration, aliénation, amentia, aveuglement, délire, déraison, divagation, égarement, extravagance, folie	aberration, alienation, amentia, blindness, delirium, unreason, rambling, bewilderment, insanity, extravagance, lunacy, madness
Chinese	Sino-Tibetan	1.3 billon	失智 (Shī zhi)	dementia, lose+wisdom	痴呆 (Chīdāi)	crazy, foolish, mad, silly, stupid+trance
Norwegian	North Germanic/Nordic	5.3 million	demens	dementia	aldersdemens, senil demens, glemsk, surrete, slov, fraværende, slovsinn	old age dementia, senile dementia, forgetful, confused, blunt/dull, absent, lethargic (dull + mind)
Russian	Slavic	160 million	слабоумие, деменция	weak-mindedness, insanity, acquired weak-mindedness, insanity, infatuation, mindlessness, confusion	слабоумие, сумасшествие, приобретенное слабоумие, помешательство, увлечение, безумие	imbecility, feeble-mindedness, amentia, dotage, fatuity
Swahili	Bantu	100 million	no word for dementia	-	upungufu wa akili, hammazo, chizi, mwehu, kichaa, matatizo ya akili, ana shida ya akili	does not have a brain, unintelligent, faulty brain, mad, crazy, mental problems
Urdu	Indo-Aryan	70 million	ڈیمنشیا	dementia	یاداش کھونا (yaadash khona), پاگل (pagal), دماغی الجھن (dimaghi uljhan), دولت میں تبدیلی (rawai mai tabdeeli)	memory loss, mad, brain confusion, changes in behaviour

We do so by deriving from Saussure's dyadic description of sign (consisting of a signifier and signified) and social constructivist (Berger & Luckmann, 1966; Kress, 2010) approaches to semiotics. The words we use are culturally available semiotic resources (Kress, 2010), instruments whose purpose is to communicate the speakers' choices within a specific linguistic and cultural tradition. We look at the available examples of terminology that surround dementia as a semiotic resource that conveys different messages, meanings and values.

According to the hypothesis of linguistic relativity, also (misleadingly) labelled as the 'Sapir–Whorf hypothesis', the structure of a given language influences both the cognition and the worldview of the speaker (Leavitt, 2010). This means that our perception of phenomena such as dementia could be relative to the language we speak. In addition to the very structure of the language, the vocabulary we use constructs our reality and shapes how we think about the world, too (Bartlett & O'Connor, 2010).

Take, for example, how the word 'therapy'[1] is used within the context of the prevention and treatment of dementia. Singing, listening to music, gardening, playing an instrument, visiting an art gallery, swimming, weight-training, cycling, walking, and other regular leisure activities all become 'therapies' in the context of people with dementia. Over the years, the word 'therapy' has come to dominate the understanding of the actions and lives of people with dementia. Even when a person with dementia creates a protest banner, it is likely to be described by others in terms of 'art therapy' rather than an act of citizenship (Bartlett, 2015) (the nature of art as therapy is discussed by Dowlen and Fleetwood-Smith in Chapter 10, and another example – of people's stories being described as therapy – is considered by Kindell and colleagues in Chapter 9). The reasons for this are complex. In part, it comes down to the fact that medical discourse, along with a/the biomedical pathologising gaze and objectification for purposes of scientific inquiry, has long played a central role in diminishing the status of people who live with dementia (see also Fletcher's discussion of the biopolitics of dementia in Chapter 2).

In other languages, different words and phrases are available to describe aspects of everyday life. Such words reflect the values of that culture and, in turn, help to construct the reality of living in that society. For example, in Norwegian, the term 'friluftsliv' (outdoor life) denotes a commitment to and appreciation of the time spent in nature, both enjoying the weather and in spite of it. In Japanese, the term 'shinrin-yoku' (forest bathing) is used to describe the practice of walking, viewing, and just simply spending time in a forest atmosphere (Martin et al., 2019, p. 8). Examples show how language and culture overlap - words and phrases evolve to capture cultural values and priorities. This has implications for not only care practices (Martin et al., 2019) but also a person's status and potential role in society (Bartlett & O'Connor, 2010). Knowing and appreciating a language and all its idioms is a sign of belonging to the culture in which it is spoken. It is why someone with dementia with an immigrant background might 'dread losing the language' of their adopted country (Demensplan 2025, 2020, p. 18) – they know language is an integral part of social identity and status.

Sharing a language is linked to status and community, and it involves sharing meanings. If these meanings are not understood by others (i.e., carers), then one's sense of community is at stake (Puumala & Shindo, 2021, p. 752). The way we express ourselves through language remains a 'central component of commonality and is a key medium of affirming and claiming belonging' (Puumala & Shindo, 2021, p. 751). For example, a multilingual person with dementia with diminishing language skills may develop a new way of communicating with family members to express a desire and make themselves understood. Language is based on social conventions, a characteristic that implies the inevitability of speaking and writing about anything that concerns a minority from a position of the majority. This is, of course, true of all languages.

When multiple languages are spoken in a care context, or if translators are used to facilitate communication, it may not be possible to get 'to know the person' and provide truly 'person-centred care', as miscommunication and misunderstanding become key features of interactions. For example, interactions with multilingual persons with dementia might become complex as the person may revert to speaking only their primary language as the condition progresses (Khan, 2011).

Making sense of the world plays a central role in all our lives. While our main tool for meaning-making is language, it is only the tip of the iceberg. Other semiotic resources such as multimodal codes (pre-linguistic and pictorial, for example), customs, tradition, pragmatics and cultural memory (Lotman, 1990), to name a few, affect both our linguistic experiences and our understanding of the world. By exploring how language and culture shape our perception of dementia, we also examine how these meanings influence people's attitudes and behaviours.

Use of the term dementia globally

Romance languages

The term dementia can be traced back to the 13th century when it was used to refer to a lack of judgment and imagination (Assal, 2019, p. 119). It was first introduced to the medical community in the 18th century (around 1797) by a French physician and one of the founders of modern psychiatry, Philippe Pinel. At the time, Pinel was also considered to be an alienist (aliéniste, fr.), which was a common term for physicians who worked with people with mental disorders. Considering that the word alienation has connotations of isolation and estrangement in different languages, it is possible to trace how dementia, along with mental disorders, has been constructed as otherness. Dementia, too, has been marginalised by means of language and, as such, is part of a wider depreciative lexicon of mental disorders, one that has historically been considerably institutionalised, even in well-intentioned contexts of care.

Pinel described dementia as extreme incorrectness, thoughtlessness and wild abnormalities, a mental derangement commonly characterised by rebellious and raging movement, passionate feelings and a rapid succession of ideas in the affected person's mind (Pinel, 1806). Both biomedical and everyday language related to dementia evolved in France too, and has over time included words such as 'aliénation' (alienation), 'aveuglement' (blindness), 'délire' (delirium), 'déraison' (unreason), 'divagation' (rambling), 'égarement' (bewilderment), 'extravagance', 'folie' (lunacy, madness) and various others. Due to colonial heritage, dementia-related French vocabulary is used across the world. Various semiotic resources, connotations, values and attitudes were exported along with terminology – for example, many languages (see Table 4.1) have borrowed the word for dementia (and its meanings) from French, an addition to the aforementioned alienation and delirium, to name a few. Due to this, discussions and understandings of dementia are almost as dominant and influential as those coming from the Anglophone world, with an ever-growing body of available literature, and will not be the main focus of this chapter.

However, an interesting recent example of the use of the word dementia as a metaphor (one of the core semiotic resources) and as a diagnosis in public discourse comes from Italian, which belongs to the same language group as French. With around 85 million speakers, it is also one of the most widely used languages. The instance demonstrates how the term still retains a rather negative connotation in certain parts of the world and is misused by officials and the media in public discourse to evoke fear. In his text 'War and (Senile) Dementia'[3], published just days after the Russian invasion of Ukraine in February 2022, Franco Bifo Berardi poses a question: 'Can humanity save itself from the murderous violence of the demented and agonised Western, Russian and European brains?' (Berardi, 2022b). The Italian philosopher here refers to two 'white brains', those of current American and Russian presidents Joseph Biden and Vladimir Putin, that have 'entered a furious crisis of senile dementia', and further describes these supposedly dementia-affected brains as characterised by impotent anger, and a decline in psychic energy, cognitive efficiency and strength. Such an assertion considerably resonates with Pinel's description of dementia as a mental derangement characterised by raging and passionate feelings.

The derogatory use of the term dementia in common parlance goes well beyond this example and the language in question. However, such high-profile utterances do more than serve as innocent metaphors – they further stigmatise already vulnerable people who live with dementia by adding to depreciative, demeaning connotations.

Chinese

Our focus in this section is on how the Chinese language and culture have defined and characterised dementia over the years. We start in ancient China and the formation of traditional Chinese Medicine (TCM). According to Liu et al. (2012), the earliest description of dementia can be traced back to a classic ancient text written over 2000 years ago – 'The Yellow Emperor's Classic' – widely considered the origin of traditional Chinese medicine. In this text, dementia was described as an 'insufficiency of Qi, a flowing energy; and the loss of memory was attributed to Qi moving in the wrong direction' (Liu et al., 2012, p. 2948). Formal descriptions of dementia then developed in the Han Dynasty (202 BC–220 AD). During this period, derogatory terms were used, and dementia was defined as 'Chi Dai' (痴呆),

which means 'stupid' and 'retarded'. Stupid is commonly defined in English as not having the ability to absorb ideas readily; it can also mean showing a lack of good sense or judgment. Others used the term 'Shi Zhi' (失智, loss of wisdom) to denote dementia. In the Song Dynasty, dementia was named 'Chi' (痴, being excessively obsessed with something; capricious and stupid). In the Yuan Dynasty, the term 'Dai' (呆, being stunned, slow mind and stupid) was used to describe dementia (Liu et al., 2012). Historically, then, in Chinese, dementia has been understood in an entirely negative way.

In modern China, descriptions of dementia have changed from those bearing completely derogatory meanings to more biomedically informed understandings. Medical and healthcare professionals in China are now more likely to understand dementia as a brain disease than an individual character flaw. This shift in meaning shows how omnipresent the biomedical pathologising gaze has been, and continues to be, in the field of dementia. That said, the situation in China (and Chinese) deserves special attention when analysing the meanings of dementia as 'traditional Chinese medicine and biomedicine co-exist' and the culture has a long history of dealing with competing political ideologies (Zhang et al, 2018). Thus, it is important to trace the roots of the term dementia back to Ancient China and the origins of traditional Chinese medicine.

Norwegian

The aforementioned Nordic model, among other things, aims to destigmatise the views and approaches to dementia and those directly affected by it, as well as to create a more dementia-friendly society (Demensplan 2025, 2020, p. 46) – unfortunately, these ideals are not inherent in the Norwegian language (see Table 4.1); it seems that the lexicon still has some catching up to do. This is the cultural and academic context in which this chapter is written. It is also a setting in which we can observe how the change in perception of phenomena affects cultural norms and customs, and vice versa.

Norway was one of the first countries in the world to present a comprehensive strategy for the provision of services to people with dementia (Demensplan 2025, 2020). The third and most recent iteration of a 5-year plan came out in late 2020 and opens with an interestingly worded goal: 'Our goal is that no one should experience the same as the participant in the [focus group for Demensplan 2025] input meeting: to be thrown into an uncertainty and go into the fog ('gå inn i tåkeheimen') when the disease strikes' (Bent Høie, Former Minister of Health and Care Services of Norway, Demensplan 2025, 2020, p. 5). The statement was made in the context of the value of receiving a timely diagnosis and appropriate post-diagnostic support, but it shows how dementia is seen as an attack on one's way of life.

The most commonly used term is a direct translation of the word dementia, 'demens'. This is partly due to a sustained (most of all cultural) effort to transform the rapidly aging society into a more inclusive one. Such practices have allowed for the eradication of stigmatising language over time – a work that is still in progress. For example, pejorative signifiers such as 'åndssvak' (mentally retarded) are gradually being replaced with terms that can also be used to signify persons who neither live with dementia, nor with mental illness, such as 'hen er litt åndsfraværende' (they are a bit absentminded), 'hen lever i sin egen verden' (they live in their own world). Such descriptions may be less harsh, but they are still othering – persons with dementia ('they') are positioned as a separate group, different from the rest of the population (Canales, 2000).

Back to the former minister Høie's metaphor ('going into the fog when a disease strikes') – it is not an isolated example of experiences of dementia being described in terms of presence, absence and disappearance. Other expressions and synonyms, such as 'ikke helt med' (not quite there/not quite good with it), 'fraværende' (absent) and 'åndsfraværende' (spirit/mind + absent), also propose a perception of dementia that is characterised by a loss. This loss can be a loss of sharpness ('sløv', blunt or dull or 'sløvsinn', meaning lethargic, of dull mind), spirit, presence or ultimately personhood.

Russian and other Slavic languages

Studies on the prevalence or the therapy of dementia are rare or non-existent in Russia (Kostev & Osina, 2020). Similarly, reliable statistics regarding the number of patients with dementia in Russia are lacking, and so is a national plan to combat dementia (Pishchikova, 2017). According to the Alzheimer's Association, over 1.5 million people live with dementia in Russia (Alzheimer's Association Russia, 2022). However, this might be an underestimation, considering that many people receive a diagnosis at later stages or do not receive it at all (Granina, 2017).

Russian and other Slavic languages commonly use the word dementia to refer to the condition: 'деме́нция' (Russian), 'деменція' (Ukrainian), 'деменција' (Bosnian, Northern Macedonian, Serbian), 'demencija' (Croatian, Montenegrin, Slovenian, Slovak) or 'demencja' (Polish). However, prior to the standardisation of medical terminology to include direct translation, dementia was described in other terms. These terms remain synonymous today.

For example, the other most widely used word for dementia in Russian is слабоумие (weak-mindedness). Other synonymous words include 'сумасшествие' (madness, distraction, craziness), 'приобретенное слабоумие' (acquired weak-mindedness, dementia), 'помешательство' (insanity, lunacy), 'увлечение' (passion, enthusiasm, rage), 'безумие' (mindlessness), 'идиотия' (idiocy) and 'имбецильность' (imbecility). The condition is described as a breakdown of mental functions and is otherwise informally referred to as 'старческий маразм', meaning old person craziness. The Ukrainian word for dementia, 'божевілля', literally translates as god's freedom or will and refers to madness and frenzy, while the South-Slavic synonym for dementia, 'izlapelost' signifies staleness, depletedness or exhaustion.

One striking example of how dementia-related language remains stigmatising despite the standardisation of medical literature and its attempts to become more inclusive is an article published in a popular Russian online media outlet in 2017, titled 'В квартире с монстром: болезнь превращает стариков в чудовищ' (In an

Apartment with a Monster: the Disease Turns Old People into Monsters) (Cikulina, 2017). This article uses semiotic resources characteristic of literary genres such as horror to describe the experiences of living with dementia from both perspectives of persons with dementia and their care partners.

The author uses the word 'dementor' to refer to a person who has dementia; a word with similar connotations in Russian to those in English: a fearsome and evil creature. 'What is just as terrible as the death of the person with dementia', writes Cikulina, 'is the horror of the disease taking life and strength from the patient's loved ones' (Cikulina, 2017). The article further paints a fear-inducing image of dementia for those unfamiliar with the condition: 'Caring for a dementor is not like caring for a person with any other serious illness: dementia often turns a person into a monster, trashing an apartment and throwing themselves at the people closest to them' (Cikulina, 2017). The author also argues for the institutionalisation of people with dementia, not for their benefit but for the benefit of their carers, by quoting one person's family member who compares a person with dementia with a vampire:

'The worst thing is not that many sick people turn into animals, smear excrement all over the apartment, destroy furniture, throw things out of the window, and try to run away from home. All these problems are solved with the help of reliable locks and space restrictions. It is scary that people with dementia try to drink all the juice from the loved ones who care for them. And it is very difficult to understand how to do it in such a way as to build psychological protection around yourself and not succumb to provocations'.

(Cikulina, 2017)

This framing of dementia experiences, as recent as in 2017, using pejorative language that denotes horrors, evil, animality and monstrosity not only stigmatises those affected by the condition but also isolates and devalues people by describing them as less-then-human and depriving them of their personhood – a feature that is not necessarily unique to the Russian language. In addition to the aforementioned, the expressions such as 'the living death' and 'the death that leaves the body behind' present people living with dementia as inhuman and echo Susan Behuniak's analysis of the social construction of people with Alzheimer's disease as zombies (Behuniak, 2011).

Swahili

Although it is impossible to count how many words exist in Swahili, many words, including those of non-Bantu origin, cover different concepts and aspects of everyday life (Zawawi, 1979; Hurskainen, 1999). There is currently no specific word in Swahili that signifies dementia. However, a few expressions with both negative and neutral connotations are used in referring to different presentations or assumptions of dementia.

A common expression for dementia is 'Upungufu wa akili' (the one who does not have a brain). The phrase is used for someone who has very significant memory problems or behaves in ways considered extreme or unusual. It is sometimes an umbrella signifier for profound mental health, cognitive or intellectual issues. 'Hamnazo' is another term with negative connotations used to refer to someone with dementia. It comes from the verb 'not having' and directly translates to someone who is not intelligent or whose brain is faulty. Other words with negative connotations include 'chizi', 'mwehu' and 'kichaa', which all translate to 'mad person' or 'crazy person'. These words with negative meanings are rarely used to describe loved ones or relatives, especially not to their hearing, except if the intention is to offend or hurt the person. They can, however, be used with close friends when joking with them.

Other expressions in Swahili used to refer to dementia or a person living with dementia include 'matatizo ya akili' (mental disorders) and 'ana shida ya akili' (has a mental disorder). In Swahili-speaking countries, as is the case in much of Africa, dementia is largely not considered or framed within the context of medical understandings by laypeople but is based on individual and communal. Framings with negative connotations often have adverse effects on people with dementia. Studies from the continent – especially regarding the framing of dementia as witchcraft or evil – have shown that attaching negative meanings to dementia can lead to the stigmatisation and devaluation of people living with dementia (see, for example, Brooke & Ojo, 2020).

On the other hand, health professionals will likely use the same terminology for dementia and intellectual or mental health challenges, as we demonstrate above. Similar to the other languages, these phrases are perceived as objective and value-free. Just like in the aforementioned modern Chinese languages, a biomedical understanding aims to supersede the view of dementia as a personal character flaw in Swahili too. This reinforces our initial claim regarding the temporal character of acceptable language related to dementia and the idea that initially preferred vocabulary is often itself replaced.

Urdu

Urdu is another language that has no specific word for dementia. This may be because dementia, for many people, is not conceived of as a distinct illness but either as a normal aspect of aging or as a severe mental problem. Intergenerational living is the norm for many households in Pakistan, and care for the elderly is usually left to the family – including managing dementia and other impairments. People are rarely diagnosed with dementia within a medical setting and thus commonly develop their own ways of making sense of different aspects of dementia and its treatment. The only word for dementia in Urdu is the English word 'dementia', or 'ڈیمنشیا' in Urdu script. There are, however, other words and expressions used in reference to different aspects of dementia or different understandings of dementia, such as 'یاداشت کھونا' (yaadash khona) meaning memory loss, 'پاگل' (pagal) meaning mad, 'دماغی الجهن' (dimaghi uljhan) meaning brain confusion, and 'رویے میں تبدیلیاں' (rawai mai tabdeeli) meaning changes in behaviour.

In situations in which people do not perceive dementia as either a medical condition in need of the healthcare system's support or as an impairment that requires reimagining and related redesigning of social and physical structures to accommodate the specific needs of those who live with it, people with dementia may find themselves continuously faced with insufficient care and unmet needs. According to our informant, as the healthcare and social welfare system continue to develop in Pakistan and scholarship on dementia becomes more accessible, it is expected that the care and provision accessible to people with dementia will also grow, both within a state-provided and a communal care system.

Conclusion

This chapter demonstrates how the meaning of dementia is constructed by means of Chinese, Swahili, Urdu, Norwegian, French, Italian, Russian and other Slavic languages and how this construction both affects and reflects the perception of dementia in these and related cultures. Semiotic analysis of language regarding dementia beyond English has revealed that meanings have changed over the years across the world, but also that meanings of *dementia* share similarities and differences, even if languages might stem from different roots. One similarity is that dementia is, or has been, described in negative and stigmatising terms; in some languages, such as Russian, the negativity is particularly strong and reflected in terms such as weak-mindedness and comparisons to monstrosity. Such perception echoes Trachtenberg and Trojanowsky's (2008) view on the word dementia, for whose eradication they argue: 'At its unkindest, it is a word without hope, which is a crucial tool when faced with a devastating illness'. One difference, on the other hand, is that in some languages, such as Urdu and Swahili, there is no word for dementia. Instead, expressions such as 'mental disorder' are used (in Chapter 3, Mason and colleagues note that people with dementia can be distressed by this general language of mental illness).

While it has not been the focus of this chapter, how dementia is spoken about and understood culturally has implications for how people with the condition are treated. Previous work has shown how in many cultures across the world the signs and symptoms of dementia are often regarded as either a normal part of the aging process or as a mystical and religious experience (Mackenzie et al., 2005). In Nigeria, for example, some people will understand dementia-type symptoms as a sign of demonic possession and/or loss of faith. People showing such symptoms are therefore chastised or punished and subject to special prayers and vigils (Mackenzie et al., 2005). Language matters then. Not only academically but also in a very real way for those who develop and live with the condition.

While language is easier to implement in professional settings such as the academic, medical and legal, in addition to Norwegian, an example from Japan suggests that such change is possible in common parlance if the state or political awareness and willingness allow for it. Namely, the word for dementia in Japanese, ' Chihō', has a negative association. 'Chi' means foolishness, and 'hō' means dumb or disoriented. It contributes to stigma and fails to show dignity and respect for people with dementia. Therefore, at the end of 2004, the Japanese government changed the word for dementia from 'Chihō' to 'Ninchishō', which means 'disease of cognition'. The government has changed all administrative terms to the new word, and the media and academic groups have also accepted the new term. In light of this, it could be argued that, at least implicitly, biomedical terminology remains symbolically preferable.

Languages are fluid and immersed in sociocultural contexts. This discussion captures vocabulary and meanings characteristic of specific temporality – hence the need to develop a critical history of language in dementia studies. Far from being innocent and value-free, languages frame how people think of everyday phenomena, and these perceptions vary across cultures and time. Finally, how we perceive a phenomenon, such as dementia, inevitably influences how we relate to persons with dementia as well as how we organise prevention and care.

Acknowledgment

We acknowledge the native speakers and professionals we spoke to about this chapter and who have helped us understand language differences.

Notes

1 Therapy comes from the Greek word therapia (healing) and denotes a treatment intended to heal or treat physical, mental or social disorders or diseases.
2 Table 1: The translations have been derived in consultations with native speakers. We additionally did a reverse translation of all words and expressions using various dictionaries and translation tools, including Google translate, Merriam-Webster and Collins dictionaries.
3 The text was originally published in Italian under the title 'Guerra & Demenza (Senile)' Berardi (2022a) in late February 2022. The quote is Andreas Petrossiants' translation for the e-flux journal, published weeks later.

References

Alzheimer's Association Russia. (2022). *Alzheimer's and Dementia in Russia*. https://www.alz.org/ru/dementia-alzheimers-russia.asp. Accessed May 25, 2022.
Assal, Frédéric. (2019). History of Dementia. In Bogousslavsky J, Boller F, Iwata M (eds.). A History of Neuropsychology. Basel: Karger. 44: 118–126. https://doi.org/10.1159/000494959.
Bartlett, Ruth. (2015). Visualising Dementia Activism: Using the Arts to Communicate Research Findings. Qualitative Research, 15 (6): 755–768.
Bartlett, Ruth, O'Connor, Deborah. (2010). Broadening the Dementia Debate: Towards Social Citizenship. London: Policy Press.
Behuniak, Susan M. (2011). The Living Dead? The Construction of People with Alzheimer's Disease as Zombies. Ageing & Society, 31 (1): 70–92. https://doi.org/10.1017/S0144686X10000693
Berardi, Franco. (2022a). Guerra & Demenza (Senile). in Not Nero Editions. https://not.neroeditions.com/guerra-demenza-senile/. Accessed June 22, 2022.
Berardi, Franco. (2022b). War and (Senile) Dementia. in e-flux Journal #125. https://www.e-flux.com/journal/125/454088/war-and-senile-dementia/. Accessed June 22, 2022.

Berger, P. L, Luckmann, T. (1966). The Social Construction of Reality: A Treatise in the Sociology of Knowledge. Garden City, NY: Anchor Books.

Brooke, J., Ojo, O. (2020). Contemporary Views on Dementia as Witchcraft in Sub-Saharan Africa: A Systematic Literature Review. Journal of Clinical Nursing, 29(1–2): 20–30. https://doi.org/10.1111/jocn.15066

Canales, Mary K. (2000). Othering: Toward an Understanding of Difference. Advances in Nursing Science, 22(4): 16–31.

Cikulina, Svetlana (Цикулина, Светлана). (2017). В квартире с монстром: болезнь превращает стариков в чудовищ. https://www.mk.ru/social/health/2017/03/14/v-kvartire-s-monstrom-bolezn-prevrashhaet-starikov-v-chudovishh.html. Accessed June 2, 2022.

Demensplan 2025. (2020). Helse-og Omsorgsdepartementet. https://www.regjeringen.no/no/dokumenter/demensplan-2025/id2788070/. Accessed June 28th, 2022.

Granina, Natalia. (2017). Маразм крепчает Скоро Россию захлестнет эпидемия слабоумия, которую никто не ждет. Lenta.ru https://lenta.ru/articles/2017/10/16/dementia/. Accessed May 28, 2022.

Hurskainen, A. (1999). SALAMA: Swahili Language Manager. Nordic Journal of African Studies, 8(2): 139–157. https://doi.org/10.53228/njas.v8i2.639

Khan, Farooq. (2011). Being Monolingual, Bilingual or Multilingual: Pros and Cons in Patients with Dementia. International Psychiatry, 8(4): 96–98.

Kostev, Karel, Osina, Galina. (2020). Treatment Patterns of Patients with All-Cause Dementia in Russia. Journal of Alzheimer's Disease Reports, 4(1): 9–14. https://doi.org/10.3233/ADR-190144

Kress, Gunther. (2010). Multimodality – A Social Semiotic Approach to Contemporary Communication. New York, NY: Routledge.

Leavitt, John Harold. (2010). Linguistic Relativities: Language Diversity and Modern Thought. Cambridge: Cambridge University Press.

Liu, Jia, Wang, Lu-ning, Tian, Jin-zhou. (2012). Recognition of Dementia in Ancient China. Neurobiology of Ageing, 33 (12). https://doi.org/10.1016/j.neurobiolaging.2012.06.019

Lotman, Yuri M. (1990). Universe of the Mind: A Semiotic Theory of Culture. London: LB. Tauris & Co Ltd.

Mackenzie, J., Bartlett, R., Downs, M. (2005). Moving towards Culturally Competent Dementia Care: Have We been Barking up the Wrong Tree?. Reviews in Clinical Gerontology, 15(1): 39–46.

Martin, C., Woods, B., Williams, S. (2019). Language and Culture in the Caregiving of People with Dementia in Care Homes – What Are the Implications for Well-being? A Scoping Review with a Welsh Perspective. Journal of Cross-Cultural Gerontology, 34(1): 67–114. https://doi.org/10.1007/s10823-018-9361-9

Pinel, Philippe. (1806). A Treatise on Insanity: In which Are Contained the Principles of a New and More Practical Nosology of Maniacal Disorders than has Yet Been Offered to the Public. Sheffield, England: W. Todd.

Pishchikova, L. (2017). The Strategy to Combat Dementia in Russia. European Psychiatry, 41: S662. https://doi.org/10.1016/j.eurpsy.2017.01.1120

Puumala, Eeva, Reiko Shindo. (2021). Exploring the Links between Language, Everyday Citizenship, and Community. Citizenship Studies, 25(6): 739–755. https://doi.org/10.1080/13621025.2021.1968696

Trachtenberg, Don, Trojanowsky, John. (2008). Dementia. A Word to be Forgotten. Archives of Neurology, 65 (5): 593–595.

Young, Holly, Sundberg, Minna. (2015). A Language Family Tree – in Pictures. In Guardian. https://www.theguardian.com/education/gallery/2015/jan/23/a-language-family-tree-in-pictures. Accessed May 15, 2022.

Zawawi, S. (1979). Loan Words and Their Effect on the Classification of Swahili Nominals. Leiden: Brill Archive.

Zhang, Min, Chang, Yu-Ping, Liu, Yu Jin, Gao, Ling, Porock, Davina. (2018). Burden and Strain among Familial Caregivers of Patients with Dementia in China. Issues in Mental Health Nursing, 39(5): 427–432.

5 Literary dementia studies

From managing estrangement to imaginatively reconceptualising forgetfulness

Heike Hartung

Introduction: Narrating age from the *Bildungsroman* to the dementia narrative

In the early 1990s, the 'coming of age of literary gerontology' was announced by humanities scholar Anne M. Wyatt-Brown. With this term, she described work that was initially based mainly in the US-American humanities, which encompassed studies of artistic creativity in later life, psychoanalytic and biographical approaches to the ageing of artists, analyses of forms of the life review in literature as well as studies of the impact of the emotions on the ageing process in literary representation (Wyatt-Brown 1990, Wyatt-Brown and Rossen 1993). If the 'coming of age' chronicled the beginnings of this approach to ageing discourses in literature studies in the late twentieth century, by the early 2020s literary gerontology may be seen to have reached 'maturity'.

Even if one should be wary of using developmental categories modelled on the lifecourse, which tend to 'naturalise' a trajectory of progress and decline that has been criticised in Age Studies (Gullette 2004) (see the introductory chapter of this volume for such a critique), they can be useful to explore historical dimensions of discourses of old age and dementia critically. Developmental age categories have frequently been used to conceptualise literary history, for instance in the English context, where the novel of the late seventeenth and eighteenth centuries has been described by many literary scholars as the genre's unruly youth, characterised by a multitude of disparate forms such as the sermon, letter-writing or romance. During the eighteenth and early nineteenth century, the novel has left these stages of childhood and early youth, reaching maturity with the emergence of psychological realism (Eagleton 2005: 94). In his posthumous study *On Late Style*, Edward Said makes the connection between literary historical discourse and individual biography explicit, when he distinguishes three stages for both, first, the time of 'beginning', 'birth' and 'origin', second, the 'time from birth to youth, reproductive generation, maturity' and third, 'the last or late period of life, the decay of the body' (2006: 4–6). Said identifies the middle period with 'the *bildungsroman* or novel of education' (5).

As I have argued in more detail elsewhere, the *Bildungsroman* is the genre of the novel that makes the process of ageing itself its central concern. Whereas the

DOI: 10.4324/9781003290353-8

genre was more interested in depictions of youth and early adulthood when it was first conceived, this shifted to later stages of the life course. Literary narratives of dementia, which emerged in many European literature from the 1980s onwards, can be seen as both questioning the limits of processes of *Bildung* and ageing, but also as narrative constructions that expand notions of development beyond chronological narration (Hartung 2016: 170–220).

Originating in the late eighteenth century in Germany, with Johann Wolfgang Goethe's *Wilhelm Meisters Lehrjahre* (1795/96) as its model text, the *Bildungsroman* has been associated with modernity, mobility and interiority (Moretti 2000). Age categories were affected by the shift to modern societies when the life span became a more stable, even predictable, standardised category during the eighteenth century. This was expressed in exemplary form in the German literary genre of the *Bildungsroman*, which 'dramatized the fight of the developing individual against the social programs into which he (never she) was supposed to grow' (Kohli 1986: 293). Whereas the central protagonists of the *Bildungsroman* in its earliest forms were indeed White, middle-class young men, the genre has been appropriated since then to include more diverse subjects. From the perspectives of feminist and gender studies, the 'female' *Bildungsroman* was shown to have accompanied the 'male model' from the genre's beginnings, even if notions of female formation have remained much more restricted than the male version during the eighteenth and nineteenth centuries (Hirsch 1979, Bannet 1991). Twentieth- and twenty-first century rewritings of the *Bildungsroman* have opened up its model of human development, which has been questioned from the various perspectives of cosmopolitanism, human rights and ethnicity (Japtok 2005, Slaughter 2007, Boes 2012).

During the twentieth century, the genre increasingly included later stages of the lifecourse, in the *Reifungsroman* that depicts middle age, specifically for women, as 'a time of discovery, liberation, and adventure' (Waxman 1990: 11), and in the *Vollendungsroman*, which extends the developmental plot into older age (Rooke 1992). Illness was already associated with the development of Goethe's protagonist Wilhelm Meister in a novel that linked physiological aspects of formation to a temporal dimension. Mortal illness is used as a comparison when Wilhelm first encounters loss in the betrayal of his first lover, while the physical intensity of this experience is compared by the narrator to the decomposition of a corpse (Goethe 1795/1995: 41). The function of illness in the classical *Bildungsroman* is thus linked in multiple ways to its representation of ageing as development. While the genre takes many different directions in the twentieth and twenty-first centuries, the focus on illness becomes central in narratives of dementia. The dementia narrative, in its concern with frail old age frequently tells stories about reaching the end of ageing (of course this might also be argued of much of the life history narrative collected or created with people who have dementia themselves; see Chapter 2 by Capstick, and Chapter 9 by Kindell and colleagues, for further discussion). I employ this descriptive term broadly to refer to autobiographical illness narratives as well as fictional texts which take mental illness in old age as their central topic. As I argue, dementia narratives may define the limits of development by narrating the end of memory and consciousness, representing the dissolution of the autonomous subject. Dementia narratives also question the boundaries of life stories and, by extension, the constituents of narrativity itself, by contesting notions of development, autonomy and personhood. In this way, narratives of dementia turn the implicit concern with illness and ageing in the classical *Bildungsroman* into the direct confrontation with the connection between both.

From dementia discourse to literary dementia studies

The emergence of the dementia narrative as a new form of narrating age from the 1980s onwards in many European languages occurred against the growing public awareness of Alzheimer's disease (AD) as a risk for more people in Western Europe and the United States that accompanied increases in longevity. The genre shifted rapidly from an early focus on autobiographical self-help manuals to a diversification of literary genres, including detective and gothic fiction. One of the earliest texts, Diana Friel McGowin's autobiographical narrative *Living in the Labyrinth: A Personal Journey through the Maze of Alzheimer's* (1993), relates her experience of early-onset Alzheimer's during the 1980s when there was hardly any public awareness of the disease, even in the medical context, so that McGowin chronicles her difficulties in finding medical help or even a provisional diagnosis. Using journey and battle metaphors typical for illness narrative, the first-person text places a strong emphasis on the continuity of the self, counteracting what McGowin perceives as the labyrinthine qualities of the disease. McGowin's narrative is a self-help manual 'from the patient's perspective' (1993: vi) intended for people in similar situations, which describes her own strategies of secrecy, distancing and self-camouflage, a text that to a certain degree 'masks disease' (Basting 2003: 89).[1]

Two early fictional approaches to dementia paint an equally grim picture of the disease, focusing primarily on the estrangement and denial that the illness can provoke. Both texts promote suicide as a 'solution' to the 'problem' of dementia. The British novelist Margaret Forster's *Have the Men Had Enough?* (1989) narrates the story of dementia from the female relatives' perspective, while the person with dementia in this novel is not given a first name. The fact that she is addressed either as 'Grandma', 'Mother' or 'Mrs McKay', by kinship relation or surname, underscores the impression that she is no longer perceived as a whole person. Her granddaughter Hannah and daughter-in-law Jenny alternate as first-person narrators, both of whom remain detached from the person with dementia, while the novel focuses mainly on gender inequalities in the care for people with dementia, revealing institutional inadequacies in dementia care in the 1980s. After Mrs McKay dies in a nursing home, Hannah records a conversation with her mother Jenny, who tells her that 'Your generation, Hannah, will have to have pro-death marches, you'll have to stop being scared to kill the old' (Forster 2004: 250). Although Hannah questions this idea, the novel seems to endorse this invocation of euthanasia as a 'solution' to the 'problem' of dementia in old age, turning the illness into a metaphor for an undifferentiated fear of oldest age. In spite of its critical analysis of gender roles in care, the novel's external view of the person with dementia leads to this ageist conclusion.

A second example is the short story 'Living Will' (1991) by the American science fiction writer Alexander Jablokov, which depicts the choice of suicide from the perspective of the person diagnosed with Alzheimer's disease. The computer specialist Roman Maitland programmes a computer with his private memories, emotional commitments and linguistic idiosyncrasies, thus creating an 'electronic brain' in order to ensure that he will kill himself when he has reached an advanced stage of Alzheimer's in order to avoid becoming a 'burden' to his wife. At the gruesome ending of the story, the computer 'guides' Roman to his anticipated choice of shooting himself. The story transfers the concept of the 'living will', which emerged in the 1970s to refer to a person's written request against life-supporting measures in the case of severe illness or disablement, to a computer programmed to fulfil the person with dementia's instructions. The text thus extends the computer metaphor for the brain, which for most of the twentieth century 'dominated much of brain research and the public understanding of mind and brain' (Borck 2012: 127), into that of the computer as a successful simulation of personhood. At the same time, the story promotes an exterior, third-person approach to dementia which represents the disease reductively as 'death-in-life' (in Chapter 11, Williamson and Jenkins debate related fears that emerging post-humanist sensibilities, which often consider agentic extension via digital technologies, risk dehumanising people with dementia).

These three early examples of dementia narratives were written during a time of little public awareness of the disease, in which negative responses of denial prevailed both in autobiographical and fictional texts. Public recognition of AD changed rapidly during the 1990s and to a degree that has been described by critical gerontologists as the 'Alzheimerisation of ageing' with reference to a differentiation of old age into a healthy, active third age to the detriment of a 'demented' fourth age of irrevocable latest-life decline (Gilleard and Higgs 2000: 40). In the twenty-first century, the 'Alzheimerization of Growing Old' (Beard 2018) has come to signify the problematic conflation of the disease with its late stages. In a quest for ever earlier diagnoses associated with the label 'mild cognitive impairment' (MCI), this has led, particularly in the United States, to a thorough medicalisation of AD (for further discussion of the rise of the 'Alzheimer movement' in the United States, see Chapter 1 by Fletcher). While biomedical research focused in the 1990s primarily on 'post-symptomatic interventions', this shifted towards a focus on early detection and prevention, transforming the cultural definition of AD from 'a brain condition, a neurochemical disturbance, to a general health condition' (Leibing 2015: 277). In the current situation of supreme attention given to AD both in medical research, diagnostics and clinical practice, while significant treatment options or even a cure remain elusive, the question is, in Rene Beard's words 'what early diagnosis means, sociologically speaking, for [people living with dementia] and the rest of us, as we age and anticipate ourselves as *future old people*' (2018: 169).

Therefore, a more personalised approach to medical research into treatments and cures for the different forms of dementia that incorporates a focus on how people with dementia and their families live with these early diagnoses is important. This is where the humanities, and literary dementia studies in particular, can step in. In the early twenty-first century, humanities research has focused on the relational aspects of dementia, for instance in Anne Davis Basting's alternative approach to narrative as performance in her writing workshops for people with dementia in the pioneering project 'TimeSlips' (Basting 2005). Empirical approaches to literature, both narrative and poetry, which establish its relevance for the care of people with dementia while remaining critical of a purely medical view, have been developed by Aagje Swinnen (2016, 2018, and also in Chapter 9), Kate de Medeiros (2011) and de Medeiros and Swinnen (2018). Furthermore, punitive illness metaphors such as the 'zombie trope' have been analysed to show how certain types of language use generate negative cultural meanings for the condition, which denigrate people living with dementia (Behuniak 2011, Zeilig 2014).

With the emergence of a variety of representations of AD and dementia in literature, film and the arts, a veritable 'cultural "dementia boom"' has set in (Swinnen and Schweda 2015: 10), which has been experienced differently in many European countries, the United States or India, which have until now been the main focus of this dementia discourse (Dowlen and Fleetwood-Smith explore this 'boom' in Chapter 10). Work in the anthropology of ageing and dementia has early on foregrounded conceptual and cultural differences (Cohen 1998, Leibing 2006, Whitehouse, Maurer and Ballenger 2000), while in recent years research in literary dementia studies has proliferated. Literary genres such as the memoir and life writing (Zimmermann 2017), detective fiction and children's literature (Falcus and Sako 2019) have been examined in book-length studies. This scholarly work illustrates the variety of perspectives on dementia that different literary genres may provide, ranging from distance to closeness to the person with dementia. They also give voice to the person with dementia and their relatives, while the professional carers' voices still remain underrepresented. Specific topics related to dementia discourse have been analysed, such as how forgetting and remembrance is affected by national histories (Krüger-Fürhoff, Schmidt and Vice 2022); in what ways gender is relevant to dementia (Hartung 2022); or how care is represented in dementia fiction (Falcus and Sako 2021). Dementia literature from different national contexts is emerging, which includes work on Indian, Canadian and German-language literature in addition to work in Anglophone literature (Nayar 2018, Vedder 2012, Goldman 2015, Dieckmann 2021, Christ forthcoming).

The growing popularity of representations of AD and dementia in the arts has not led to a complete removal of the stigma attached to the syndrome, so that there is no simple 'progress narrative' to be told from the perspective of literary dementia studies. For instance, the idea that the person with dementia ultimately becomes a burden to his or her relatives prevails as a form of ageism which may even promote what Margaret Morganroth Gullette (2011: 43) has termed 'the duty to die' in the context of debates on physician-assisted suicide. More recent dementia novels like Lisa Genova's *Still Alice* (2007) or Alice LaPlante's *Turn of Mind* (2011) can be read as variations of the 'burden topos': By foregrounding the 'height' of their protagonists' minds – in the first case a cognitive psychology professor, in the second a hand surgeon – they suggest the 'downfall' that is their 'decline' as an effect of Alzheimer's.[2]

However, even if negative representations of the person living with dementia continue to be published, the picture has become more differentiated as knowledge about the disease has increased. The exclusive association of personhood with memory and the brain, as in Jablokov's short story, has shifted to medical models promoting the brain's plasticity. More recent definitions of dementia have also redefined the 'heart-brain connection' with the result that medical interventions target 'the brain *as part of the body*' (Leibing 2015: 277). These shifts in the medical understanding of dementia show that knowledge about the illness in all its cultural implications is provisional at best, constituting what Annette Leibing has called 'knowledge in the making' (2015: 280). From the 1990s, proclaimed in the United States as 'the decade of the brain', in which the growing awareness of Alzheimer's initiated the 'personhood movement' that began to acknowledge the person with dementia as active and socially participating (Leibing 2006) to the 'recasting of the phenomenon of AD as a condition to be prevented' since the early twenty-first century, the complexities of the disease in its entanglement with the ageing process has led researchers to 'confront head-on the ontological question of what exactly is AD', raising difficulties also to distinguish 'what counts as "normal" and what as "pathological"'(Lock 2013: 2–3).

Rather than attempting to provide an outline of the developments within the dementia narrative, which has begun to proliferate within different national and cultural contexts, as the enormous output in recent years sketched above illustrates, in what follows I will analyse the Norwegian writer Linn Ullmann's recent novel *De Urolige* (2015; *Unquiet* 2019) in the context of filial narratives of paternal dementia. As a case study this text is particularly interesting in its implications for dementia discourse, since in its treatment of the father's growing forgetfulness in old age it may serve as an example for an alternative approach to dementia that is less concerned with diagnosis or medicalisation.

Even if *Unquiet* is not, strictly speaking, a dementia narrative, I read the text strategically as one, drawing on an approach employed by Gullette in her analysis of Jane Austen's novel *Emma* (1815) as a dementia narrative *avant la lettre*, in which she argues that the protagonist Emma's gentle care-taking of her forgetful father may 'provide lessons for our Alzheimer's-obsessed era' (2011: 169). What Gullette calls 'Pre-Alzheimer's nostalgia' in Austen's novel, written long before Alois Alzheimer named the condition in 1906, may be seen also as an illustration of what recent literary dementia studies have argued, namely that memory and forgetting are situated in a social and cultural context beyond the medical, and that the self is relational.

Linn Ullmann's *De Urolige* (*Unquiet*): Un-Naming dementia

Linn Ullmann's *Unquiet*, though a fictional text, is based on the Norwegian writer's autobiographical experience with her well-known parents, the Swedish filmmaker Ingmar Bergman and the Norwegian actress Liv Ullmann. In its autobiographical motivation it shares features with other filial narratives of paternal dementia, described by autobiography scholar G. Thomas Couser as a 'subset of the memoir of illness and disability', in which sons or daughters write about their parents, investigating 'their memories of growing up', while the parents – as the 'irreplaceable repositories of these memories' become 'eventually unavailable' (2021: 81).

Ullmann's novel has similarities with other literary narratives of parental dementia, such as the Austrian novelist Arno Geiger's book on his father, *Der alte König in seinem Exil* (2011; *The Old King in his Exile*, 2017), or the American drama professor Elinor Fuchs's memoir on her mother, *Making an Exit* (2005), both of which incorporate the voice of the person with dementia. Geiger uses conversations with his father, which represent August Geiger's idiosyncrasies of speech, to introduce individual chapters of his literary memoir. Fuchs similarly foregrounds the performative function of language in apparently nonsensical exchanges with her mother. In Ullmann's novel, the voice of 'the father' is incorporated in dialogue sequences, which refer to tape recordings made at an earlier stage by the narrator. These were intended for a book project on the father's old age to be written in collaboration with the daughter. The father is also present through other media like notes to the daughter, his private letters as well as the filmmaker and writer's extensive archive.

As outlined above, the approach to AD and dementia in medical research has shifted from a focus on symptoms to one of prevention without substantially changing the life quality of people living with dementia, so that early diagnosis does not make much sense from a social and cultural perspective. This question of diagnosis and medicalisation serves as my point of entry for reading Ullmann's novel as a text which not only eschews a diagnosis of dementia for the father's forgetfulness, but intentionally rejects naming itself. In the novel the main protagonists remain without names, generically called 'the girl', 'the mother', 'the father'. Ullmann, who was a literary critic in Norway before she became known internationally as a novelist, stated in an interview that the elision of central names provides her with the freedom that makes the text fiction rather than autobiography, while its form remains fragmentary (Mason 2019).

Neither using names for her characters nor employing the category of dementia for the changes in her father, Ullmann's narrator becomes self-reflexively interrogative when she refers to the series of minor strokes regarded by the father's doctor as responsible for the changes to his memory and perception: 'he no longer distinguishes between dreams (I don't know whether dreams is the right word here) and reality (I don't know whether that's the right word either). All the windows of his brain have been thrown wide open' (2020: 60). As this quotation illustrates, even in a passage where the narrator refers to a medical diagnosis, strategies of naming are immediately called into question.

Unquiet is written in six parts, in an analogy to Bach's *Cello Suite No. 5*, a musical composition important to Bergman, who used it for his last film, *Saraband*. Drawing on the *Bildungsroman* genre, the novel centres on 'the girl', who is occasionally the first-person narrator, but is also depicted from an external third-person perspective. Her frequently disturbing experience of growing up is narrated in digressive episodes, varying both spatially and temporally, and in response to her interactions with her parents. Similar to the dementia narrative, Ullmann's text raises epistemological questions of narrativity and self, which relate to the temporal structure of experience, to the (un-)reliability of narration and memory (Peeregaard 2022: 69).

The materiality of words is one of the motifs of the novel that is established in its link to memory and old age in these conversations: 'He grew older, old, he said that things went missing. "What sort of things?"/"Words. Memories"' (2020: 42). The second section of the novel, 'Spools', makes this concern with the material aspects of words and memory, with the technologies of writing, with recording and revision, its central focus. It also highlights the importance of planning the collaborative book, variously named 'the work' or 'the project' (2020: 62), which they talk about for two years before beginning, belatedly, with the recording of their conversations: 'Happiness is finding yourself in the middle of the planning phase, when everything is possible and nothing is final' (2020: 54). The focus on the materiality of words and memory, but also the idea of being 'in the middle of the planning phase', which highlights a state of 'in-between-ness' rather than (narrative) closure, provides a positive model for imagining dementia as forgetfulness rather than as a pathological state associated with loss.

While the novel jumps in time, its six parts focus on different themes and *motifs* which are repeated in several variations, similar to the musical composition to which it refers. Part I, 'Hammars Prelude', is dedicated to the island Hammars, where the girl spends her summer holidays during her childhood with the father, whose rhythms dominate and shape this place. The father's punctuality, his need for order and rejection of improvisation are so characteristic of him that his being seventeen minutes late, when daughter and father have arranged to meet for one of their recorded conversations, constitutes the first sign of change in him for the daughter, a *motif* that runs through the whole novel: 'My father came seventeen minutes late and nothing was out of the ordinary and everything had changed' (2020: 8).

In its reference to the changes in the father, his loss of words in his last illness, the originality of Ullmann's language constitutes a form of writing about dementia without naming it, which is similar to the narrative strategies Gullette describes when she reads Jane Austen's depiction of Emma's 'kind attentiveness to her father' as a representation of dementia in a time before awareness of AD (2011: 172). In Ullmann's novel, however, there is awareness of dementia and the losses with which it is associated at our contemporary moment. Section IV of the novel, 'Have Mercy on Me', opens with a quotation from Virginia Woolf's essay 'On Being Ill' (1926), which concerns the writer's necessity to coin fresh words for representing illness, depicted as a violent process: 'He is forced to coin words himself, and, taking his pain in one hand, and a lump of pure sound in the other [...], so to crush them together that a brand new word in the end drops out' (Woolf in Ullmann 2020: 238). Ullmann's novel constitutes such a process of original creation with reference to the representation of her father's illness. In her narrator's self-reflexive questioning stance, scenes frequently begin with a statement of decline and loss but are then turned into something different and new.

In one of these episodes, the narrator acknowledges the father's loss of words, envisioning the forgotten words as 'a long, sinuous trail that stretched from the stony beach, through the forest, and all the way into the rooms at Hammars' (2020: 71). This image is juxtaposed with a scene in which the father's reckless driving provides a counter-image of action and suspense to the sense of loss. Another scene opens with the estrangement of the father sometimes recognising the daughter, sometimes not. To this, the observing narrator adds the discovery of 'a third state, more perplexing than the one or the other. He often knew who I was, but doubted whether what he knew was in fact true' (2020: 254). A third passage dwells on the diminishment of space during the last conversations between father and daughter, in which the father 'says he would like to live in a three-room flat, then he says he would like to live in a one-room-flat, then he opens the door and walks into a concert hall of such impressive proportions that birds fly around inside it' (2020: 344). All these passages take the form of a movement from a recognised loss of words or diminishment of space to something different, either a 'third state' or an enlargement based on the Ullmann's original use of language.

Although the novel *Unquiet* focuses on deep old age and illness, it is not a narrative of decline, but imaginatively reconceptualises forgetfulness as part of life's 'work'. In its depiction of the father, Ullmann does not primarily focus on his exceptional status as a public persona and artist, although this is part of her story. Instead, the emphasis is much more on ritual, repetition, the rhythms of a life lived, depicting the 'choreography of ageing' as 'complex' (2020: 354). And even though the novel is unflinching in its approach to the materialities of ageing, illness and dying, it provides in its imaginative explorations of language a form of consolation beyond closure.

Concluding remarks

Alzheimer's disease and other forms of dementia are illnesses that have come to accompany the phenomenon of mass longevity in the twenty-first century. Literary engagements with the illness may provide important contexts for thinking about dementia, impacting also on the life of persons living with it. These literary treatments can offer personalised and complex narratives of illness experience, which may contrast with and question the claims to objectivity in medical narratives foregrounding symptoms of the disease. The historical trajectory of dementia narratives since the 1980s shows that these autobiographical and fictional texts respond to and are shaped by dementia discourse. In turn, they can influence the illness experience and attitudes towards it.

There is no simple progress narrative to be told about dementia narratives: both positive and negative images for the illness continue to emerge. Nevertheless, dementia narratives contribute to the debates on memory, history and the self that are important aspects of dementia discourse. Imaginative texts like Ullmann's provide new concepts and an original language for narrating illness. The self-reflexive questioning stance in Ullmann's text makes the 'choreography of ageing' visible in its complexity. Acknowledging the complexity of this imaginary engagement with dementia is a much more effective response to punitive metaphors of the disease and the persons living with it that are still part of public debates. In the strategic unnaming of 'the father' but also of his medical diagnosis, Ullmann's novel portrays his loss of memory in the context of 'the daughter's' loss of him. Much more so than the public person of the filmmaker Bergmann, the novel makes 'the father' visible as a private person, while the kinship relationship complicates the temporal and spatial web of ageing, memory and forgetfulness in this oblique dementia narrative. My reading of *Unquiet* suggests that there is 'hope' in the potentially positive impact of such writing on contemporary attitudes towards the illness through the very act of 'un-naming' dementia.

Notes

1 For a detailed analysis of the genre of Alzheimer's life writing, which proposes a trajectory from linear to more fragmentary narration in response to 'shifting power structures' towards the inclusion of patients' voices, see Zimmermann (2017: 96ff).
2 Similar connections have been made in the case of public intellectuals, where the image of the downfall from mental heights has been used, for instance, with the writer and philosopher Iris Murdoch in Britain or the professor of rhetorics Walter Jens in Germany. See also Hartung (2022: 183).

References

Bannet, Eve Tavor, (1991), 'Rewriting the Social Text: The Female *Bildungsroman* in Eighteenth-Century England,' in James Hardin (ed.), *Reflection and Action: Essays on the Bildungsroman*. Columbia: South Carolina University Press, 195–227.
Basting, Anne Davis, (2003), 'Looking back from Loss: Views of the Self in Alzheimer's Disease,' *Journal of Aging Studies* 17: 87–99.
Basting, Anne Davis, (2005), 'Dementia and the Performance of the Self,' in Carrie Sandahl and Philip Auslander (eds.), *Bodies in Commotion. Disability and Performance*. Ann Arbor: University of Michigan Press, 202–213.
Beard, Renee, (2018), 'The Alzheimerization of Growing Old in America,' in Harm-Peter Zimmermann (ed.), *Kulturen der Sorge. Wie unsere Gesellschaft ein Leben mit Demenz ermöglichen kann*. Frankfurt: Campus, 163–173.
Behuniak, Susan M. (2011), 'The Living Dead? The Construction of People with Alzheimer's Disease as Zombies,' *Ageing & Society* 31: 70–92.
Boes, Tobias, (2012), *Formative Fictions: Nationalism, Cosmopolitanism, and the Bildungsroman*. Ithaca: Cornell University Press.
Borck, Cornelius, (2012), 'Toys Are Us. Models and Metaphors in Brain Research,' in Suparna Choudhury and Jan Slaby (eds.), *Critical Neuroscience: A Handbook of Social and Cultural Contexts in Neuroscience*. Oxford: Blackwell, 113–133.
Christ, Susanne K. (forthcoming), *Fictions of Dementia. Narrative Modes of Presenting Dementia in Anglophone Novels*. Berlin: De Gruyter.
Cohen, Lawrence, (1998), *No Aging in India. Alzheimer's, the Bad Family, and Other Modern Things*. Berkeley: University of California Press.
Couser, Thomas G., (2021), *The Work of Life Writing: Essays and Lectures*. New York: Routledge.
de Medeiros, Kate, (2011), 'Self Stories in Older Age: Crafting Identities Using Small Moments from the Past,' *American Studies/Amerikastudien* 56 (1): 103–122.
de Medeiros, Kate and Aagje Swinnen, (2018). '"Play" and people living with dementia: A humanities-based inquiry of *TimeSlips* and the Alzheimer's Poetry Project. *The Gerontologist* 58(2), 261–269.

Dieckmann, Letizia, (2021), *Vergessen Erzählen. Demenzdarstellungen in der deutschsprachigen Gegenwartsliteratur*. Bielefeld: Transcript.

Eagleton, Terry, (2005), *The English Novel*. Oxford: Blackwell.

Falcus, Sarah and Katsura Sako, eds. (2019), *Contemporary Narratives of Dementia: Ethics, Ageing, Politics*. New York, London: Routledge.

Falcus, Sarah and Katsura Sako, eds. (2021), *Contemporary Narratives of Ageing, Illness, Care*. New York, London: Routledge.

Forster, Margaret, (2004), *Have the Men Had Enough?* 1989. London: Vintage.

Gilleard, Christopher and Paul Higgs, (2000), *Cultures of Ageing. Self, Citizen and the Body*. Harlow: Pearson.

Goethe, Johann Wolfgang von, (1995), *Wilhelm Meister's Apprenticeship*. 1795. Ed. and transl. Eric A. Blackall, Victor Lange. *The Collected Works*, Volume 9. Princeton: Princeton University Press.

Goldman, Marlene, (2015), 'Purging the World of the Whore and the Horror. Gothic and Apocalyptic Portrayals of Dementia in Canadian Fiction,' in Aagje Swinnen and Mark Schweda (eds.), *Popularizing Dementia. Public Expressions and Representations of Forgetfulness*. Bielefeld: Transcript, 69–88.

Gullette, Margaret Morganroth, (2004), *Aged by Culture*. Chicago: The University of Chicago Press.

Gullette, Margaret Morganroth, (2011), *Agewise. Fighting the New Ageism in America*. Chicago: The University of Chicago Press.

Hartung, Heike, (2016), *Ageing, Gender, and Illness in Anglophone Literature: Narrating Age in the Bildungsroman*. New York: Routledge.

Hartung, Heike, (2022), 'Illness memoirs, ageing masculinities and care: The "son's book of the father",' in H. Hartung, Rüdiger Kunow and Matthew Sweney (eds.), *Ageing Masculinities, Alzheimer's and Dementia Narratives*. London: Bloomsbury, 179–195.

Hirsch, Marianne, (1979), 'The Novel of Formation as Genre: Between Great Expectations and Lost Illusions,' *Genre* 12: 293–311.

Jablokov, Alexander, (1991) 'Living Will,' in *The Breath of Suspension*. New York: Avon Books, 58–79.

Japtok, Martin, (2005), *Growing Up Ethnic: Nationalism and the Bildungsroman in African American and Jewish American Fiction*. Iowa City: University of Iowa Press.

Kohli, Martin, (1986), 'The World We Forgot: A Historical Review of the Life Course,' in Victor M. Marshall (ed.), *Later Life. The Social Psychology of Aging*. Beverly Hills: SAGE, 271–303.

Krüger-Fürhoff, Irmela Marei, Nina Schmidt and Sue Vice, eds. (2022), *The Politics of Dementia. Forgetting and Remembering the Violent Past in Literature, Film and Graphic Narratives*. Berlin, De Gruyter.

Leibing, Annette, (2006), 'Divided Gazes: Alzheimer's Disease, the Person Within, and Death in Life,' in Annette Leibing, Lawrence Cohen (eds.), *Thinking about Dementia. Culture, Loss, and the Anthropology of Senility*. New Brunswick: Rutgers University Press, 240–268.

Leibing, Annette, (2015), 'Dementia in the Making. Early Detection and the Body/Brain in Alzheimer's disease,' in Aagje Swinnen and Mark Schweda (eds.), *Popularizing Dementia. Public Expressions and Representations of Forgetfulness*. Bielefeld: Transcript, 275–294.

Lock, Margaret, (2013), *The Alzheimer Conundrum. Entanglements of Dementia and Aging*. Princeton: Princeton University Press.

Mason, Wyatt, (2019), '"I don't Want my Writing to be Charming" – Feature of Linn Ullmann' *New York Times Magazine*, Jan 10th, available online: https://www.nytimes.
com/2019/01/10/magazine/linn-ullmann-unquiet.html

McGowin, Diana Friel, (1993), *Living in the Labyrinth. A Personal Journey through the
Maze of Alzheimer's*. San Francisco: Elder Books.

Moretti, Franco, (2000), *The Way of the World. The Bildungsroman in European Culture*.
London: Verso, 2nd edition.

Nayar, Pramod K. (2018), 'Dementia in Recent Indian Fiction in English,' in Tess Magi-
ness (ed.), *Dementia and Literature. Interdisciplinary Perspectives*. London: Routledge,
148–159.

Peeregaard, Bettina, (2022), 'Despair of Self: Strategies of Seeing and Becoming in Linn
Ullmann's *De urolige*,' *Skandinavian Studies* 94 (1): 67–88.

Rooke, Constance, (1992), 'Old Age in Contemporary Fiction: A New Paradigm of Hope,'
in Tomas R. Cole, David D. Van Tassell and Robert Kastenbaum, (eds.), *Handbook of the
Humanities and Aging*. New York: Springer, 241–257.

Said, Edward W. (2006), *On Late Style. Music and Literature against the Grain*. New York:
Vintage.

Slaughter, Joseph R. (2007), *Human Rights, Inc.: The World Novel, Narrative Form, and
International Law*. New York: Fordham University Press.

Swinnen, Aagje, (2016), 'Healing words: Critical inquiry of poetry interventions in dementia care,' *Dementia 15*(6): 1377–1404.

Swinnen, Aagje and Mark Schweda, eds. (2015), *Popularizing Dementia. Public Expressions and Representations of Forgetfulness*. Bielefeld: Transcript.

Ullmann, Linn, (2020), *Unquiet*, transl. Thilo Reinhard, London: Penguin.

Vedder, Ulrike, (2012), 'Erzählen vom Verfall: Alzheimer und Demenz in der Gegenwartsliteratur,' *Zeitschrift für Germanistik* 2: 274–289.

Waxman, Barbara Frey, (1990), *From the Hearth to the Open Road. A Feminist Study of
Aging in Contemporary Literature*. New York: Greenwood.

Whitehouse, Peter J., Konrad Maurer and Jesse F. Ballenger, eds. (2000), *Concepts of Alzheimer's Disease. Biological, Clinical, and Cultural Perspectives*. Baltimore: The Johns
Hopkins University Press.

Wyatt-Brown, Anne M. (1990), 'The Coming of Age of Literary Gerontology,' *Journal of
Aging Studies* 4 (3): 299–315.

Wyatt-Brown, Anne M. and Janice Rossen (eds.) (1993), *Aging and Gender in Literature:
Studies in Creativity*. Charlottesville: University Press of Virginia.

Zeilig, Hannah, (2014), 'Dementia as a Cultural Metaphor,' *The Gerontologist* 54 (2):
258–267.

Zimmermann, Martina, (2017), *The Poetics and Politics of Alzheimer's Disease Life-
Writing*. Cham: Palgrave Macmillan.

Part III
Intersectionalities

6 Gender awareness and feminist approaches in dementia studies

Ann Therese Lotherington

Introduction

Feminist approaches are critical. They explore inequality, oppression and power dynamics to enable conceptual or social transformation. They recognise gender, race, ethnicity, class, sexual orientation and other differentiating categories as intertwined in ongoing processes of becoming of individuals and societies. Hence, understanding such complexity is a paramount demand to critical research aiming at changing the disproportional effects of privileges, dis/advantages and oppression throughout the world.

Despite the importance age and dementia have for the dynamical changes of people's lives and living conditions, and as organising principles in society, these categories are rarely found in feminist studies, whilst dementia studies suffer from a feminist deficit. The chapter picks up on this paradox, and, along three tracks, explores the potential feminist approaches might have for critical dementia studies. The first section recognises how gender awareness has revealed dementia as a feminised field. The second section discusses how intersectionality as the currently most prominent feminist approach is emerging in dementia studies. The third section promotes feminist posthumanist theory as a particularly promising way forward for critical dementia studies.

Dementia – A feminised field

Dementia care, dementia policy and dementia research still tend to refer to dementia and dementia-related issues in a non-gendered language (Bartlett et al. 2018; Sourial et al. 2020). People with dementia, family carers, care staff, and care facilities, all appear as essentialist categories populated with unified objects that might be treated in the same way. As it does not take the complexity of dementia experiences into account, this practice obscures a world of differences that matter, produces stereotypes and stigma and conceals oppressive structures. Fortunately, a demand for gender awareness is gaining momentum, and it is now widely recognised that women are disproportionately afflicted by dementia in different ways:

- The prevalence rate is higher among women than men, partly because age is a risk factor and women live longer than men, partly due to sex differences in

DOI: 10.4324/9781003290353-10

hormones, particularly how the reduction in oestrogen production affects brain function, but also other biologically and bodily sex differences that might affect brain health differently (Mosconi, 2020), and partly because a risk factor can be related to socio-economic status, and women, particularly older women, in general have lower socio-economic status than men (Sourial et al. 2020).

- Women are more often than men underdiagnosed, inter alia, because women retain their verbal abilities longer than men, despite similar brain damage (Mosconi, 2020).
- Men benefit more from dementia care and dementia care policies than women (Sourial et al. 2020).
- Women more than men take on responsibilities as carers for their loved ones with dementia, which is good for men as they might live longer at home. On the other hand, the burden on female carers makes them vulnerable to negative health outcomes, such as depression (Pillemer et al. 2018).
- Formal home- and residential home care is almost only conducted by women (Alzheimer's Disease International, 2015).

Hence, dementia might rightly be described as a feminised field. This was evident in a global research review published in 2015 (Alzheimer's Disease International, 2015) and in a scoping review published in 2018 (Bartlett et al., 2018). The two reviews conclude that the research in the field has a bias towards studies of care, both formal and informal. Only a few research papers were about gendered experiences with a life with dementia, including the effects of dementia diagnosis on femininity and masculinity. Wiersma et al. (2022) present a recent example of the importance of the two reviews' point. By taking the perspective of women living with dementia, they demonstrated the effects of their perspective to produce new knowledge. They found a range of responses in women's descriptions of their own experiences, from traditional gendered caregiver roles, via the importance of family relations in general and their role as mothers in particular, to the advantage and strength of being raised as a woman compared to being raised as a man with all the demands on men to be strong and independent, to the disadvantage of being treated differently as a woman, for example in healthcare encounters, and finally to the finding that not only did women see themselves as strong and resilient in all aspects of life, but they also described themselves as having become stronger after the dementia diagnosis. These findings are not necessarily generalizable, as they are drawn from a small sample study, but they do underscore the important point that life with dementia is not one thing but an effect of a range of intersecting conditions.

A curious observation derived from Bartlett et al. (2018) is that even if we know that women outnumber men as carers, more studies were conducted with male carers. The arguments for studying men as carers were related to their minority status. The researchers showed a greater interest in learning about men's lives and their ways of caring just because they were so few. This is a legitimate argument as there is little knowledge about men as carers, and gender sensitivity obviously also applies to men. However, if women's caring responsibilities are considered so common that there is no need for new knowledge about them, the research community itself becomes part of the problem of producing oppressive effects.

Regardless of the knowledge about higher burden on women in most aspects of dementia, little research on how to change the situation for the better is conducted. Also, little is done on the effects of existing gender norms in society related to how formal health care receives and treats women and men who ask for support. However, one example is a study on women and men who cared for their spouses with early onset Alzheimer's disease (Lotherington et al. 2018). This study found that traditional gender norms not only distributed the level of support disproportionally by gender, but also that the public healthcare system in general was highly gendered with oppressive effects on women. For example, a memory clinic was openly more sympathetic to male than female carers' needs. Men were supposed to have a legitimate need for help because no one would expect men to be able to care for a wife with a dementia. On the other hand, women in the same situation were expected to be strong and manage on her own. One woman was even told that she had to remember that as a married woman she had some duties to fulfil and stand by, as she once had promised by vowing 'I do!'. The article concludes that such systematic patterns of gendered encounters within the healthcare system calls for societal change and a renewal of the feminist slogan 'The personal is political!', as the personal experiences of oppressive treatment cannot be deemed an individual responsibility.

Gender awareness is important but a double-edged sword. On the one hand, to recognise gender differences in lived experiences and care enable new understandings of dementia and the pursuance of necessary changes. On the other hand, it is a danger. If the differences are acted upon as natural and acceptable, then stereotyping, stigmatising and oppression might be maintained and even enhanced, like we saw in the example from the memory clinic. Gender awareness is, therefore, not enough. The differences must be analysed in terms of power and inequality and be acted upon accordingly (Sandberg, 2018). Gender as a binary relating to women and men only is also a dangerous path. First, gender is more than women and men, and second, gender is only one differentiating category that matters.

Intersectionality as a thinking tool

In 1989 Kimberlé Crenshaw coined the concept 'intersectionality' as a structural and dynamic understanding of power in which sexism and racism intersect and produce the conditions for Black women's lives (Crenshaw, 1989). Her conceptualisation grew out of a long history of Black feminists' theorising of Black women's lives. The theorising concerned discrimination against Black women, not only as women and not only as Black, but as women and Black at the same time as something different from being either women or Black. In line with a feminist life course approach, intersectionality opens for historical, political and economic contexts, and includes in the analysis long-term effects of intersecting dimensions of power (Utz & Nordmeyer, 2007). The approach grew in popularity among Crenshaw's contemporary and subsequent feminist colleagues across disciplines.

For many academics, intersectionality became even an analytical tool for under-standing identity on an individual level, and not structural discrimination. Increas-ingly also other differentiating mechanisms than gender and race were enrolled, and intersectionality became a general feminist approach in analysis of the complexity of identity and identity formation. This development has been critiqued for fading the Black feminist genesis and consequently for concealing Black women, and for its non-structural understanding of subjectivity and identity (Cooper, 2015). This is not to claim that Black women always should be subjects of study or that certain categories always should be privileged, but that the foundational idea should be integral to its further development, namely that 'intersectionality reflects a commit-ment neither to subjects nor to identities per se but, rather, to marking and mapping the production and contingency of both' (Carbado, 2013: 815). Then, the object of study becomes what the intersection of various power dimensions produces regard-ing inequality, discrimination and subordination. Part of this is also to include the top of power hierarchies, such as whiteness, maleness and heteronormativity, and analyse how these are produced (Carbado, 2013) (in Chapter 7, Ludwin discusses heteronormativity in the representation of people – and particularly women – with dementia in cultural products). In particular, the inclusion of whiteness and male-ness as part of the production of a social category, even if unarticulated, is one way to ground the analysis in the heritage from Black feminist thought (see Chapter 8, by Roche and colleagues, regarding the developing attentiveness to race in de-mentia studies and the dangers that this can generate when poorly conceived and executed).

Within dementia studies the intersection of gender and other differentiating power mechanisms is rare but not completely absent (Sandberg, 2018). Intersec-tional analysis might start with gender but does not a priori privilege gender or take gender or other categories for granted (Calasanti, 1996). What differentiating power mechanism(s) are foregrounded depend on the focus of the study. Critical dementia studies might analyse how dementia intersects with gender and either produce *gender* or *life with dementia* differently. In her theoretical exploration of gender and dementia, Sandberg (2018) provides several examples of how the gender/dementia intersection *produces gender differently*. She points out how the dehumanising discourse of dementia as loss of personhood and bodily control is intertwined with loss of gender such that it is not possible to distinguish between being a person and being gendered. However, this gender/dementia intersection is rarely questioned or made explicit. Sandberg describes how inappropriate gender appearances often is understood in biological and cognitive terms as loss, at the same time as the abject dementia body is related to inappropriate gender appear-ance. Consequently, to maintain personhood in dementia, orderly femininity and masculinity must be restored, often through appropriate clothing, hair styles and manicure (for women) and shaving (for men). The case demonstrates how the in-tersection of dementia and gender on the one hand produces abject individuals, and on the other hand, how well intended care interventions to maintain person-hood produce femininities and masculinities that might restrict behaviour and po-tentially suppress emancipatory changes in life. Alternatively, in a feminist lens non-conforming gender appearances enabled through dementia might be under-stood as expressions of relief of pressure to perform in certain gendered ways, with certain sexual preferences, hence, as disruptions of oppressive gendered structures, not only between men and women but also among and between cis and LGBQ-TIA+ people.

With a research focus on life with dementia, the gender/dementia intersection and other intersecting power structures should be part of the analysis, as different intersections *produce different experiences of dementia.* Hence, intersectional stud-ies will not take any understanding of life with dementia for granted but enquire into how the meaning of dementia might be produced and shift according to gender, class, race, sexuality, etc., and analyse how various forms of interconnectedness of the power mechanisms might preserve or dissolve oppressive, marginalising prac-tices. (In Chapter 2, Capstick also points out the need for a historical dimension in intersectional studies of dementia).

In her study, Wendy Hulko (2009) points out how the (still) dominating nega-tive understanding of life with dementia (dementia as loss), described as for ex-ample 'hell on earth', 'slow death', 'gruesome torture' and 'loss of self', has been grounded in studies of privileged people's experiences with early-stage dementia (for a discussion of the impact of such terms on people living with dementia, see Mason and colleagues in Chapter 3). To account for other narratives and to explore the diversity and heterogeneity of life with dementia, Hulko applied an intersec-tional, power approach. She involved participants with different gender, ethnic, class and 'racial' identities, and with a variation in severeness of the illness to delve into 'insider' experiences of life with dementia, which she, in line with Alzheimer's Disease International (2015) and Bartlett et al. (2018), had identified as a deficit within dementia studies. Hulko found that a variety of experiences of life with dementia, from very negative ('hellish') to dismissing its significance ('not a big deal'), were related to the participants' degree of privilege. Whilst the multiply privileged people confirmed the dominating negative understanding, the multiply marginalised people did not worry much about it but described their lives with dementia as a different way of life one must relate to.

Implicit in Hulko's conclusion is a critique of the neo-liberal understanding of normalcy and the 'desirable citizen' (Jenkins, 2017: 1487) that defines dementia as decay and produces people with a dementia as abject (Latimer, 2018, Sandberg, 2018). However, dementia is not one thing, it multiplies in time and space, and a shared identity as people with dementia does neither equal the same identity nor the same experiences of a life with dementia, as a deviant sameness. This was also evident in the already mentioned study by Wiersma et al.'s (2022). Consequently, dementia research should take such new knowledge seriously, critically dismantle dominating dementia narratives and their oppressive effects, and propose prosper-ing alternatives.

Intersectionality is at its best when applied according to the original idea, to analyse how structural power dynamics produce conditions for life differently. It is 'a conceptual and analytic tool for thinking about operations of power' (Cooper, 2015: 405), and herein lie promises for understanding the complexity in dementia experiences, not as individualised and personal but as societally constituted in time and space.

When, on the other hand, intersectionality is applied to understanding subjectivity or personal identity, at least two problems arise: the first concerns research methods and methodology, the second individualisation and what it means to be a human.

The first problem – methods and methodology – relates to the understanding that identities/subjectivities are not fixed. Categories (gender, race, class etc.) do not pre-exist but are dynamically constituted in intersections. Consequently, study participants cannot be selected and included according to fixed categories. The question is, therefore, how the research design alternatively should be developed to ensure the inclusion of all relevant differentiating mechanisms in the analysis. There is no quick fix to this problem as categorical thinking is deeply rooted in Western scientific thought and language, and hence fundamental for standard scientific methods. However, the increasing tendency to conduct transdisciplinary research, and experimenting with new methods and exploring other ways of knowledge production, such as art-based research and indigenous knowledge, might point towards new possible methodological paths.

The second problem with applying intersectionality to analysis of subjectivity and personal identity relates to individualisation and the troubled relationship with the neoliberal understanding of what it means to be a human. What counts as 'human' in neoliberalism is a coherent, rational, self-contained, autonomous, male self that constitutes the norm for normality. Everyone else is different and less human. There remains no room for people with dementia here, 'except as carriers of loss' (Quinn and Blandon, 2020: 25). We do not need more research telling us that dementia equals loss, rather, we need the subversive potential of critical feminist dementia research to produce new, liberating knowledge for people with dementia and other non-conforming individuals. Intersectionality applied as a structural power lens is one option, feminist posthumanist theory another. Feminist posthumanist theory endorses the fundamental ideas of intersectionality and acknowledges the importance of understanding the complexity of phenomena but takes the thinking in a somewhat different direction. The proposition of feminist posthumanist theory as a promising path for critical dementia studies is, therefore, not to contrast intersectionality but to demonstrate what this approach might offer.

Feminist posthumanist theory

The 'humanist' in feminist posthumanist theory refers to the legacy of Western thinking from Aristotle, via Enlightenment to the modern episteme, in which the human is privileged as the knower and the doer, and, as already described, not just anybody but a human with characteristics excluding most living beings from the category 'human' and his privileges. Critical dementia studies approaches, such as personhood, selfhood, human rights and citizenship, dissociate from this exclusionary comprehension. They challenge the narrow understanding of the human, widen the category, and include people with dementia as human knowers and doers.

These approaches have gained substantial influence on how we think of people living with dementia, how a life with dementia might be lived, and how dementia care should be organised and conducted. However, despite this commendable work, the approaches remain human-centred and contingent of the epistemic humanist heritage that order people according to compliance with the norm for normality. For example, if we claim that people with dementia can do what those without the diagnosis can, like being agentic or struggle for their cause, we measure people with dementia against the current societal norm for normality. Even critical approaches might, therefore, be part of the problem of exclusion and discrimination they aim to diminish (Jenkins, 2017) (see also Williamson and Jenkins' debate on the relative merits of human rights-based approaches and posthumanism in Chapter 11). The 'post' in feminist posthumanist theory is a response to this problem. Through critical interrogation of the implications of human-centred thinking for our understanding of phenomena and proposals for different ways forward, we might de-centre the human and direct our research beyond humanism.

According to Braidotti (2022), feminism is a precursor of what she calls the posthuman turn in research, and feminist posthumanist theory might be traced back to the 1980's. The approach has since advanced widely across academic fields (Braidotti, 2015), but not much towards dementia studies. The application and advancement of the approach within dementia studies are still in an initial stage (Quinn & Blandon, 2020), and less conspicuous as *feminist* posthumanist theory than as posthumanist theory. Despite the importance of feminism for the development of posthuman theory, mainstream posthumanism tend to neglect feminism. Nonetheless, because of its transformative power, the 'feminist' in feminist posthumanist theory is crucial to hold on to. A feminist approach is concerned with emancipation of the marginalised and asks whether a practice is liberating for the marginalised, rather than asking whether their status is, or should be, equal to some normative standard, such as the 'human'. In the end, feminist knowledge production advances understandings of how inequality, oppression, and power dynamics come into being and operate, and how it all could be different, including how we may live in difference together. Because feminist posthumanist theory understands the world as on-going intra-actions of becoming, everything might be different from how it appears. Consequently, nothing should be taken for granted but questioned. This is demanding in practice, as the requirement is potentially limitless, but questioning what is taken for granted should be the gold standard of our thinking.

The person in this approach is not a coherent, rational, individualised pre-existing 'human' but an agent that emerges through and as part of entanglements as results of intra-action (Barad, 2007). Barad prefers 'intra-action' to 'inter-action', because 'inter-action' refers to actions between separate agents. 'Intra-action' on the other hand, allows for understanding individuals as entangled and becoming: 'Individuals do not preexist their interactions; rather, individuals emerge through and as part of their entangled intra-relating' (Barad, 2007: IX). What is entangled will vary in time and space, and different thinkers might privilege different things and name the entangled agents differently. Important contributions are the Cyborg (Haraway, 1985/2004), Assemblages (Deleuze & Guattari, 2001), the Body

Multiple (Mol, 2002), Symbiont (Jenkins, 2017) and Human-more-than-human in time-space (Barad, 2007).

However, posthumanist theory is not one coherent, grand theory, but a set of theoretical propositions. The mentioned thinkers might, therefore, disagree on various propositions despite operating within a shared ontology of becoming (Bergstedt, 2021). They have in common their concern with entanglements, and the rejection of the Cartesian, individualised understanding of the person as distinctively separated in binaries such as woman/man, young/old, sick/healthy and dualistic separation of phenomena such as nature/culture, public/private, knower/known, us/them, human/animal, and, not least important in critical dementia studies, mind/body. In contrast, no category is seen as fixed or clean but performed or enacted (Mol, 2002) differently in different entanglements in which humans, non-human animals and matter intra-act. It is not 'either-or' but 'both-and'. Being entangled means to lack independent, self-contained existence. No one/thing can be or act independent of others. All phenomena, including individuals, become as effects of intra-actions. All are mutually co-constituted and interdependent but who and what constitutes the interdependence varies in time and space. Consequently, the object of research is the *becoming* of phenomena, that is, what the entanglements produce, not the *being* of individuals, self, or other phenomena. This is a non-representational way of thinking with consequences for research, because when the world is understood as on-going intra-actions of becoming, it cannot be represented but must be enquired as it unfolds (Alaimo & Hekman, 2008; Thrift 2008; Vannini, 2015). More important than reporting on what happened in the past (representation), what happens now and what might become (non-representation) concerns posthumanist research. Each encounter holds the potential for new beginnings. The ontology of becoming (Bergstedt, 2021) and the entangled understanding of phenomena, including individuals, are what makes posthumanist theory promising for critical dementia studies (Jenkins, 2017), and feminist posthumanist theory even more so, as emancipation of the marginalised and transformation of oppressive structures, not the least gendered power structures, are paramount of feminist analysis.

With this approach, also a life with dementia is understood as on-going intra-actions, and cognition is understood beyond the individual, emerging in and through the intra-actions. What dementia might be under what circumstances, and how a life with dementia might be lived, are not defined a priori, or taken for granted (Ursin & Lotherington, 2018). Dementia is not analysed as a property pertaining to the individual but as an effect of the configurations that shapes everyday life. Sometimes the illness might dominate and take over, other times it means little or nothing. The illness becomes just another intra-acting agent, not the one causing specific and predictable effects as described in biomedical definitions of dementia. Whether dementia comes to the fore as afflictive and devastating depends on the entanglements, not the diagnosed person.

In addition to the human-more-than-human intra-actions, *time and space* are crucial for how and what the illness-agent does and what it might mean. Hence, how everyday life recursively and relationally is configured, how and when human-more-than-human agents take part in the configurations, and what effects the configurations might have for whom, are of core interest in feminist posthumanist research. What a woman, a man, a trans person etc. living with dementia can and cannot do, and how they might live their gendered lives, are not taken for granted or decided a priori but enquired and understood as effects of intra-action. The conditions for life and possibilities for new beginnings are shaped in and through the entanglements in which also life course take part as one agent.

To exemplify this, the following examples are feminist posthumanist reinterpretations of two intersectional studies. The first example is drawn from already mentioned Wiersma et al. (2022), the second from O'Connor et al. (2010).

Wiersma et al. (2022) illustrate the point that one life course experience, namely women's traditional caring roles, may produce different effects depending on entanglements with dementia and other agents. When 'before' and 'now' were active agents in these women's stories about life with dementia, the effects of the entanglements were burden and stress, because suddenly, they were the ones in need of care who no longer could live up to their and others' expectations to them as carers for others. On the other hand, when 'men' were active agents in the stories, the entanglement produced strength. The women saw themselves as better to handle a life with dementia than men, because their caring experiences and long history of supporting others' coping needs could be transferred to own coping strategies. Men did not have such experiences as part of their life course, rather, they had been cared for when needed. Also, according to these women, the masculinised demand on men to be strong during the entire life course became a disadvantage for them when dementia became part of their entangled lives. Weakness, then, would mean loss of masculinity. Hence, to analyse stories like these with pre-defined gendered understandings of the subject would not only maintain gender stereotypes, but also miss the opportunity to see differently and see different things.

The second example is drawn from O'Connor et al. (2010), who demonstrate the heterogeneous character of experiences with dementia. They did a case study of an aboriginal woman diagnosed with young-onset dementia, positioned in a socioeconomic non-privileged situation, living with a same-sex partner. Most notably, this study showed how the entanglement of dementia with ethnicity and cultural heritage produced emancipatory effects, such as artistic creativity, connectivity to ancestors and peacefulness. However, her unconventional relationship to dementia entangled with young age produced disregard from the environment of the afflicting effects of the illness. Even her loved ones and healthcare people had a hard time understanding that she had a dementia and hence a need for support and care to cope with the difficulties that, with dementia, had taken part in the constitution of everyday life. A fixed understanding of dementia and its supposed effects preserved marginalisation and threatened an otherwise creative and prosperous life with dementia. This negative effect was amplified as the environment did not recognise her female partner, neither as a partner, nor as one also in need of care and support as a partner to a woman with dementia. Here a heteronormative standard produced oppressive practices that with other understandings might have become different.

In feminist posthumanist research the centre of attention shifts from individuals' actions and relations between coherent human subjects, to examining the entanglements and their effects; from practitioners to *practices*, from the doing subjects to the *doings* (Vannini, 2015). Consequently, events replace individuals as objects of enquiry, as events encompass both relations and doings that might be changed. In this way we may understand how conditions for life, such as sexism, racism, ageism and ableism, come about, but also the potentials made available for living in difference together, fighting oppression and developing policies for change.

Anchored in a history of feminist research ethics, feminist posthumanist research seeks to meet a continued need for affirmative, relational and caring ethics (Braidotti, 2022). This should be the norm in critical dementia studies. A guiding principle for *the researcher* should be to leave the position as a supposed abstract agent outside of the phenomenon of study to become an active part inside of it, making the relations between the knower and the known entangled (Barad, 2003; Haraway, 1997). It is not that the researcher ceases to be researcher and the person living with dementia no longer lives with dementia, and the two collapse into one and become each other, but that the knowledge produced as an effect of the entanglements in which the two agents take part neither can be traced back to the researcher nor to the person living with dementia. The knowledge is co-produced and the significance of the distinction between those with and those without a dementia diminishes or is even ruled out in certain time-spaces. The researcher as an individual does not produce knowledge *about* persons living with dementia or *with* them, which both maintain an undesirable distinction between 'us' and 'them', but the entanglement of researcher, person living with dementia and other human-more-than-human agents produces new knowledge. The majority, 'us without dementia', is also questioned and included. How do 'we' affect the process of marginalising 'them'? This is an important question in feminist research, as it makes the researcher vulnerable alongside the already defined vulnerable research participants. And vulnerability, like all other phenomena, should be scrutinised. Who the vulnerable is, and what produces vulnerability, depends on the entanglements in time-space. As Donna Haraway points out: '(…) no one is standard or ill fitted in all communities of practice' (1997: 38). Hence, who is 'ill-fitted' and when, is an empirical question. In some practices the ill-fitted ones might well be those deemed healthy whereas those with a dementia might fit completely in.

Challenging the balance and shift between fitted and ill-fitted, is one way to leave the traditional researcher position and become part of the phenomenon of study. To do this demands not only engagement with new research approaches, such as creative and playful practices, appealing to senses other than the rational ones, but also courage to let go of own self-consciousness, engage with the discomfort, and embrace the complexity and nuances of the situation. For example, in multi-sensorial artistic entanglements of art materials, music, dance, women and men with dementia, artists and researchers, we as researchers might feel ill-fitted but at the same time become knowers in new, entangled ways. The affectivity and connectivity such entanglements produce, might enable value to the art of life and open for understandings of different possibilities for prosperous lives with dementia (Lukic & Lotherington, 2019; Mittner, 2021).

Because feminist posthumanist theory challenges the core elements in modern thinking, such as the foundational normative subject of neoliberalism, categorical thinking, being-ontology, and concepts, language and metaphors of science, the approach might be demanding. Both mainstream research and own scientific legacy might oppose the attempts at doing research differently. However, the knowledge we produce with feminist posthumanist theory might enable a desire for dementia, not as loss, but as new possibilities in life, and hence, ways to live and thrive in difference together (Latimer, 2018). The approach is, therefore, a promising path forward for critical dementia studies.

References

Alaimo, S. & Hekman, S. (eds.) 2008. *Material Feminisms*. Bloomington & Indianapolis: Indiana University Press.

Alzheimer's Disease International. 2015. *Women and Dementia. A Global Research Review*, Alzheimer's Disease International, London.

Barad, K. 2003. Posthumanist Performativity: Toward an Understanding of How Matter Comes to Matter. *Signs: Journal of Women in Culture and Society*, 28 (3), 801–831.

Barad, K. 2007. *Meeting the Universe Halfway. Quantum Physics and the Entanglement of Matter and Meaning*. Durham & London: Duke University Press.

Bartlett, R., Gjernes, T., Lotherington, A.T., & Obstefelder, A. 2018. Gender, Citizenship and Dementia Care: A Scoping Review of Studies to Inform Policy and Future Research. *Health and Social Care in the Community*, 26(1), 14–26. https://doi.org/10.1111/hsc.12340

Bergstedt, B. 2021. The Ontology of Becoming: To Research and Become with the World. *Education Science*, 11, 491. https://doi.org/10.3390/edusci11090491

Braidotti, R. 2015. Posthuman Feminist Theory. *The Oxford Handbook of Feminist Theory*, 673–698. https://doi.org/10.1093/oxfordhb/9780199328581.013.35

Braidotti, R. 2022. *Posthuman Feminism*. Cambridge: Polity Press.

Calasanti, T.M. 1996. Incorporating Diversity: Meaning, Levels of Research, and Implications for Theory. *The Gerontologist*, 36(2), 147–156. https://doi.org/10.1093/geront/36.2.147

Carbado, D.W. 2013. Colorblind Intersectionality. *Signs: Journal of Women in Culture and Society*, 38(4), 811–845.

Cooper, B. 2015. Intersectionality. *The Oxford Handbook of Feminist Theory*, 385–406. https://doi.org/10.1093/oxfordhb/9780199328581.013.20

Crenshaw, K. 1989. Demarginalizing the Intersection of Race and Sex: A Black Feminist Critique of Antidiscrimination Doctrine, Feminist Theory and Antiracist Politics. *University of Chicago Legal Forum*, 1(8). http://chicagounbound.uchicago.edu/uclf/vol1989/iss1/8

Deleuze, G., and Guattari, F. 2001. *A Thousand Plateaus: Capitalism and Schizophrenia*. London: Athlone Press.

Haraway, D. 1997. *Modest_Witness@Second_Millennium. FemaleMan©_Meets_Onco-Mouse*. London: Routledge.

Haraway, D., 1985/2004. A Manifesto for Cyborgs: Science, Technology, and Socialist Feminism in the 1980s, in Haraway, D. *The Haraway Reader*. New York and London: Routledge, 7–46.

Hulko, W. 2009. From 'Not a Big Deal' to 'Hellish': Experiences of Older People with Dementia. *Journal of Ageing Studies*, 23(3), 131–144. https://doi.org/10.1016/j.jaging.2007.11.002

Jenkins, N. 2017. No Substitute for Human Touch? Towards a Critically Posthumanist Approach to Dementia Care. *Ageing and Society*, 37, 7, 1484–1498. https://doi.org/10.1017/S0144686X16000453

Latimer, J. 2018. Repelling Neoliberal World-making? How the Ageing-Dementia Relation Is Reassembling the Social. *The Sociological Review Monographs*, 66(4), 832–856. https://doi.org/10.1177/0038026118777422

Lotherington, A.T., Obstfelder, A., & Ursin, G. 2018. The Personal Is Political Yet Again: Bringing Struggles between Gender Equality and Gendered Next of Kin onto the Feminist Agenda. *NORA – Nordic Journal of Feminist and Gender Research*, 26(2), 129–141. https://doi.org/10.1080/08038740.2018.1461131

Lukic, D. & Lotherington, A.T. 2019. Fighting Symbolic Violence through Artistic Encounters: Searching for Feminist Answers to the Question of Life and Death with Dementia. In Vaittinen, T. and Confortini, C.C. (Eds.). *Gender, Global Health and Violence*. London: Rowman & Littlefield International, 117–139.

Mittner, L. 2021. Resonating Moments. Exploring Socio-material Connectivity through Artistic Encounters with People Living with Dementia. *Dementia*, 21 (1), 304–315. https://doi.org/10.1177/14713012211039816

Mol, A. 2002. *The Body Multiple: Ontology in Medical Practice*. Durham and London: Duke University Press.

Mosconi, L. 2020. *The XX Brain*. New York: Penguin Random House LLC.

O'Connor; D., Phinney, A. & Hulco, W. 2010. Dementia at the Intersections: A Unique Case Study Exploring Social Location. *Journal of Aging Studies*, 24 (1), 30–39.

Pillemer, S., Davis, J. & Tremont, G. (2018) Gender Effects on Components of Burden and Depression among Dementia Caregivers. *Ageing & Mental Health*, 22 (9), 1162–1167.

Quinn, J. & Blandon, C. 2020. *Lifelong Learning and Dementia: A Posthumanist Perspective*. United Kingdom: Palgrave Pivot. https://doi.org/10.1007/978-3-030-42231-8

Sandberg, L.J. 2018. Dementia and the Gender Trouble?: Theorising Dementia, Gendered Subjectivity and Embodiment. *Journal of Aging Studies*, 45, 25–31. https://doi.org/10.1016/j.jaging.2018.01.004

Sourial, N., Arsenault-Lapierre, G., Margo-Dermer, E., Henein, M. & Vedel, I. 2020. Sex Differences in the Management of Persons with Dementia Following a Subnational Primary Care Policy Intervention. *International Journal for Equity in Health*, 19, 175. https://doi.org/10.1186/s12939-020-01285-2

Thrift, N. 2008. *Non-Representational Theory: Space, Politics, Affect*. New York: Routledge.

Ursin, G. and Lotherington, A.T. 2018. Citizenship as Distributed Achievements: Shaping New Conditions for an Everyday Life with Dementia. *Scandinavian Journal of Disability Studies*.20(1), 62–71.

Utz, R.L. and Nordmeyer, K. 2007. Feminism, Aging, and the Life Course Perspective. *The Gerontologist*, 47(5), 705–716. https://doi.org/10.1093/geront/47.5.705

Vannini, P. 2015. Non-Representational Methodologies: An Introduction. In Vannini, P. (Ed.) *Non-Representational Methodologies. Re-Envisioning Research*. London and New York: Routledge, 1–18.

Wiersma, E.C., Harvey, D., & Caffery, P. 2022. 'I'm Still the Queen and I'm Still on My Throne…': Women's Reflections on Gender and Living with Dementia. *Journal of Women & Aging*, https://doi.org/10.1080/08952841.2022.2054656

7 'On my good days, I can [...] almost pass for a normal person'

Reading The film *Still Alice* using the conceptual lens of heteronormativity

Katherine Ludwin

Introduction

Seven years ago, I wrote a blog post titled *Heteronormativity and Dementia: What's the Relevance?* (Ludwin, 2016). In it, I sketched out the case for drawing on the concept of heteronormativity – which describes the privileging of a specific, narrow version of heterosexuality – in the context of dementia studies. I argued that although people experience access to services, for example, differently depending on social markers related to family, dementia is nevertheless largely treated and portrayed as a category unmarked by social location. Historically, there has been an *almost* seamless assumption in the majority of practice, research and popular representation that sexuality, marital status and family composition are not relevant or significant to understanding what it is like to live with a dementia diagnosis. Importantly, over the last decade or so, an emergent body of research, practice and representation has begun to explicitly trouble this concerning disregard, pointing out, for example, how heterosexuality is routinely assumed in the context of dementia care and how people living with dementia who identify outside of heterosexuality often experience, or live in fear of experiencing, real-world discrimination in the course of accessing or trying to access key services (Di Lorito et al, 2021; Peel and McDaid, 2015; Price, 2012). In the context of important work such as this, focused on the experiences of marginalised sexualities, heteronormativity has often been used without much definition and/or interchangeably with homophobia and heterosexism.[1] However, since around the mid-2010s, there has been some acknowledgement within the critical dementia studies that heteronormativity is a distinct concept which can be drawn on to offer additional insights and understanding. This signifies a notable shift in the field as the important organising influence of a specific narrow version of heterosexuality across many aspects of society is acknowledged as having potential implications in relation to the experience of living with dementia. In 2016, Richard Ward and Elizabeth Price made a case for 'opening up a radical critical space at the margins of mainstream dementia studies', advocating for engagement with the concept of – amongst other critical theory concepts – heteronormativity. Interestingly, the term has remained largely undefined in terms of what it practically means or looks like, and this is returned to later in the chapter. In my blog post I suggested, as Ward and Price (2016) have done, that the

DOI: 10.4324/9781003290353-11

concept of heteronormativity held generative potential for helping to understand how a complex mediation of sexuality, gender and intimate life operated in relation to dementia. As far as I know there is currently no published work that draws on heteronormativity, as I define it in this chapter, as a conceptual tool for understanding representations of dementia in relation to norms of family and intimacy.

This chapter builds on and develops the argument I set forth in my blog post, offering an analysis of the film *Still Alice* (2014) which is based on the Lisa Genova (2007) novel of the same name, to demonstrate the utility of the concept of heteronormativity to the project of critical dementia studies. The film adaptation was written and directed by Richard Glatzer and Wash Westmoreland, a married couple who were approached to take on the adaptation when Glatzer was newly diagnosed with amyotrophic lateral sclerosis (ALS), a progressive nervous system disease. My analysis here takes place in the context of a growing body of work that, over the last two decades, has increasingly turned to an exploration of film – and other cultural products – to build an argument about how dementia is constructed. In 2009, Basting argued that the majority of cultural products related to dementia failed to engage in critical representation; as such, rather than resisting stigmatisation they largely reinforced it. Since then, others have demonstrated how portrayals of dementia overwhelmingly perpetuate and construct negative ideas about what it means to live with dementia, which can result in real-word damage for those living with a diagnosis (Behuniak, 2010). In parallel, deconstructing depictions of dementia in mainstream representation can help us to understand the extent to which, and ways in which, aspects of dementia that tend to be understood pathologically are often socially produced. There is an opportunity for the production of more thoughtful, nuanced engagement on the part of those seeking to represent aspects of dementia in their work.

The reason for focusing on the film *Still Alice* is that, although it has *been* subjected to some critical analysis, this is relatively sparse and has primarily focused on the portrayal of the diagnostic trajectory and how this is experienced; the manifestation of norms related to family and intimacy have not – to my knowledge – been considered in depth. The potential for exploring the ways in which *Still Alice* might perpetuate normative representations about dementia related to family and intimate life was touched on by Andrea Capstick et al. (2014), who reference the definition of heteronormativity employed in this chapter in relation to a sequence of films in the noughties which all centred on heterosexual, white, middle-class couples.[2] However, their work was primarily focused on inaccuracies related to the trajectory of the condition and the discord between the portrayal in the film and the realities of life for the large majority of people living with a diagnosis. As they suggest, prevailing narratives of the experiences of diagnosis have the power to perpetuate normative assumptions, a point which Annemarie Goldstein Jutel (2019: 66) also links to social location:

...there are here matters of class and of heteronormativity that are captured in the dominant diagnostic narrative motifs, and which, with only a few exceptions [...] leave numerous models for experience and illness and the medical encounter unexplored.

Sarah Falcus (2014) argues, in relation to the book, which she analyses in depth, *Still Alice* 'is such a popular and widely praised depiction of Alzheimer's disease that it is important to analyse its representation of Alzheimer's and ageing'. This is an argument that relates equally well to the film adaptation. A popular filmic representation which may influence mainstream thinking and understanding related to dementia warrants in-depth analysis in order to understand and challenge how this might inform public debate and discussion which may impact the everyday lives of those living with the condition.

It may, at first reflection, seem a strange choice to focus a consideration of normative heterosexuality on a film which is the embodiment of these norms as it depicts the lives of a solidly middle-class, white, heterosexual couple. Why not focus on a film, such as *Supernova* (2020), that *queers* the narrative in some regard and provides representations of people who live with dementia existing outside of heterosexual norms? Here – and I will return to this in greater detail later in the chapter – I am influenced by social thinkers emphasising the importance of paying attention to the 'centre' (those on the supposed privileged inside) as well as the 'margins' as a strategy to directly challenge the position that heterosexuality occupies as *the* normal, natural and organic sexuality. As Nira Yuval-Davis (1993) and others have pointed out, we must explicitly consider heterosexuality because challenging the naturalised status of hegemonic identities requires an analysis of them; this is my undertaking in this chapter. As well as paying attention to representations of those on the margins, it is useful to interrogate those that appear to be perpetuating normativity as a strategy to unsettle and call into question the assumptions upon which this is based.

I contend that paying attention to unsettling the normative core in the context of dementia is important for several reasons. The 'big society' style of political ideology that promotes minimal state support relies on the social arrangements of informal care that heteronormativity encompasses. It is therefore in the state's interests to perpetuate this ideal as a way to minimise the role of welfare support. Furthermore, the default 'person with dementia' is – as a microcosm of wider society – seen to be functioning, or trying to function, within the bounds of normative heterosexuality (hence very few depictions otherwise in mainstream representation). Without an exploration of experiences and representations of those on the supposed 'inside', the idea that there is a normal core of people who are not marked by normative heterosexuality – and for whom it somehow 'works' – is perpetuated and the 'inside'/'outside' binary remains unsettled, leaving the power hierarchies mediated through it under challenged. The act of unsettling the binary problematises the supposed normal, opening up space for an exploration of a range of familial set-ups. This, of course, is critical for understanding the lived experiences of those with dementia who – in the real world – live in as vast an array of family and intimate set-ups as there are. (The sanitisation and conventionalisation of the assumed life stories of people living with dementia is also a theme in Chapter 2, by

Capstick.) In this chapter, I argue that *Still Alice* works hard to shore up normative heterosexuality and, in doing so, simultaneously reveals its fragility, making it a fruitful film to draw on.

The chapter now turns to define heteronormativity in its theoretical context, outlining the key features for operationalising it as an analytic lens, in order to ground the case for its utility in this context. The discussion then moves on to explore the usefulness of the concept by applying it to an analysis of the film *Still Alice*, in what I hope can act as an exemplar for how this type of analysis might be approached, before drawing to a close.

Heteronormativity

Drawing on ideas already in circulation,[3] heteronormativity (Warner, 1991) is a concept that was developed from within the overlapping fields of feminist theory, gender and queer studies. It attempts to describe the ways that ideas about what it means to live a 'normal' family life relate to different levels of social privilege and inequality. This pertains to the image of family portrayed in mainstream media and entertainment, in policy, and through everyday interactions. Lauren Barlant, Michael Warner (2000: 223) describes heteronormativity as a compelling force that should be broadly understood, discussed and problematised as a dynamic:

> … produced in almost every aspect of the forms and arrangements of social life: nationality, the state, and the law; commerce, medicine; and education; as well as in the conventions and affects of narrativity, romance and other protected spaces of culture.

The version of family privileged through these mediums is heavily constructed around heterosexual relationships meaning that people identifying as other than heterosexual tend to be under-represented, misrepresented and socially disadvantaged on multiple levels. Importantly however, it is not heterosexuality per se that is privileged, but a narrow version of heterosexual family life based around certain ideas related to gender and family, which is mono-racial (overwhelmingly white); middle class (or aspires to be); and is physically and mentally 'healthy'. In addition, and of equal importance to this normative family landscape, is the inclusion of biological children, and what that represents, which links to a central part of the analysis presented later in this chapter. (As also alluded to by Lotherington in Chapter 6, heteronormativity is one of the ways that social hierarchies of power are reproduced.)

In his 2004 text, *No Future: Queer Theory and the Death Drive*, Lee Edelman identifies reproduction as the defining feature of what, in dominant discourse, 'normal' family is taken to mean. He highlights how 'the Child' (symbolically rather than any specific individual child) is held up as an emblem of 'reproductive futurity'. For Edelman, the Child represents the normative futurity of societal structure against which the queer is juxtaposed as representing the social order's 'traumatic encounter with its own inescapable failure'. Andrew King (2021: 3) takes up Edelman's work in a consideration of how dementia is framed and points out that, whilst Edelman links the Child to heterosexual futurity with the potential to 'illustrate both life's potential, but also its limits', 'we might also ask (which Edelman does not) what of the Old, or the Frail, or the Person with Dementia? Where does the symbolic Older Person stand in this futurological social order?'

In the context of this work dementia can be taken as posing a significant threat to the heteronormative order of things, and King draws on the earlier work of Linn Sandberg and Barbara Marshall (2017: 5) who write that disability 'as a threat to successful aging futures figures most clearly in the case of dementia'. King, Sandberg and Marshall all identify heterosexuality as being linked – in mainstream discourse – with 'successful aging futures', qualifying that 'heterosexuality needs to be accompanied by able-bodiedness and able-mindedness to produce visions of successful aging future' (Sandberg and Marshall, 2017: 5). In order to successfully age within dominant heteronormative arrangements, it is necessary to follow the normative life-course sequence; 'the Child becomes the Adult, reproduces and then dies' (King, 2021: 3).

Importantly, understanding heterosexuality and normative expectations related to social roles and life-course expectations that work to shore it up requires a consideration of gender because 'the hetero/homo binary makes no sense without the existence of gender divisions' (Jackson, 1999: 163; see also Richardson, 1996). Indeed, in my own research related to this issue (Ludwin, 2011), I found that ideas pertaining to acceptable (hetero)sexuality appeared to be tied up with expectations about correct ways of 'doing gender' (West and Zimmerman, 1987).

The persistent normalisation of a specific, narrow version of heterosexuality as organic over 'other' 'deviant' sexualities manifests in a multitude of nuanced ways, perpetually reproduced in the fabric of Western culture. Whilst the heteronormative nuclear family form has fragmented over the last several decades through increases in cohabitation, divorce rates, and single parent, single person households (Stasińska, 2018; Szlendak, 2015; Williams, 2004), it remains the much idealised and romanticised model that dominant discourse points us towards aspiring to; this is evident in relation to representations of people living with a dementia diagnosis in, amongst other mediums, popular film. The power of the heteronormative arguably lies in this fantasy rather than the actuality. Whilst the heteronormative family form appears to fragment, it remains a seductive ideal around which much of societal expectation and assumption circulates. As Sarah Ahmed (2004: 154) points out, this ideal is 'an impossible fantasy', but – importantly – one which families sit in different proximity to meaning some are more marginalised than other within its regulatory system.

Although part of its power lies in its ubiquity which makes it difficult to identify and call out, in earlier work (Ludwin, 2011) I mapped out some elastic definitions in terms of what I mean by heteronormativity. Setting out a flexible definitional framework is important precisely because heteronormativity is such an amorphous, variously used term that 'no one has done much explicit conceptual work with' (Chambers, 2007: 663). Whilst there has been some work theoretically grappling with the concept (see, for example, Herz and Johansson, 2015) as Joseph Marchia and Jamie Sommer (2019: 267) point out, since its first use in the early 1990s, an increasing amount of work uses the term heteronormativity, but without any consistent use (and often without clear definition at all); 'what', they ask, 'does heteronormativity actually mean?'. The elastic definitions, outlined below are focused on the primary features of heteronormativity as I use it here. The point of outlining these dynamics is to set out some tangible grounding points to work with when applying it in practice, assisting a move from the theory to the practice of operationalising it as a conceptual tool.

Conceptual framework

In order to develop my analysis, I watched *Still Alice* five times in total, reading the film with the below framework in mind. Drawing on the work of Lothar Mikos (2014: 414), I assumed that 'everything the camera shows us is important and significant', no matter how fleeting or seemingly irrelevant to the focus of the film. Each time I watched the film I made detailed notes capturing my initial impressions, recording how the content appeared to relate to the framework set out here. The notes became more detailed with each viewing and a consideration of how they related to or stretched this framework formed the basis for my analysis:

Defining features

- **The privileging of heterosexuality over all other sexualities:** Following the construction from the late 1800s onwards of ideas pertaining to an attainable 'normality' (Davis, 2006) and the codification and construction of sexuality as a core element of personhood and 'essence' (Foucault, 1979[1976]) heterosexuality has been consistently privileged as the 'normal' 'organic' and 'natural' sexuality.
- **The location of an 'other'** against which the norm depends for its naturalised status. The explicit presence of an individual or practice that subverts heteronormativity may work towards shoring it up by, conversely, providing the 'other' against which the norm depends for its naturalised existence (Chambers, 2007).
- **The defining of a 'normal way of life'** (Jackson, 2006a: 107): This is based on privileging of the individualised nuclear family over all other family arrangements: Specifically, in mainstream Western society, the privileging of a particular, narrow form of heterosexuality, based on the married, monogamous, heterosexual, reproductive (future producing), nuclear family, which relies on (context specific) gender roles. Physical and mental wellbeing are also cornerstones of this model. This family model has been particularly advanced as 'natural' since the start of the twentieth century.
- **The re-inscription of essentialist identity categories:** The heteronormative relies heavily on the sexuality (homo/hetero) binary as a mechanism through which norms of family are instituted. This relies on the gendering of subjects into two distinct parts (male/female) that together constitute a unit (the heteronormative couple). An analysis of heteronormativity should pay attention to

gender, to the ways in which gender and sexuality are (re)constructed, and to the 'empirical connections between them' (Jackson, 2006a).

- **The operation as part of a broader matrix of socially mediating systems:** As well as being heterosexual, the heteronormative family portrayed through dominant discourse is overwhelmingly white, middle class (or aspiring), and healthy. Therefore ideals about 'normal' family and intimate life both perpetuate and rely on, norms pertaining to race, class and the body as well as gender and sexuality. As Rosenfeld (2009: 618) puts it, 'heteronormativity, while a distinctive normative system, does not impose itself unilaterally, but interacts with other normative systems to shape self, identity, social action and moral evaluation'.

Given the focus here on examining representations of the normative core, and following in Samuel Chambers' (2007) footsteps, I am less concerned with (although not negating the importance of) bold statements of subversion that appear to agitate heteronormative processes from the supposed outside, and more concerned with the ways in which norms are worked on 'from within' and how heteronormativity might be unsettled from the inside. Such instances may be less obvious, more nuanced, and quieter than bold acts of subversion but they can perhaps be read as actions, feelings, or thoughts that in some way unsettle, reveal and weaken heteronormativity. Of particular relevance to my analysis here is *a repeated assertion and reassertion of heterosexuality* which begins to unmask normative heterosexuality as a fragile institution.

Considering *Still Alice*

The family unit is central to *Still Alice,* a film which is punctuated and hung together in relation to family interactions and tensions as much as in relation to the progression of Alice's Alzheimer's disease. Although at one point Alice says that memories of making friends are amongst her most 'treasured possessions', we never see anything related to friendships portrayed in the film; the film is dominated by scenes between nuclear family members. The shadow of Alice's childhood (nuclear) family hangs in the background as we find out, during an early appointment with her neurologist, that Alice's mother and sister died in a car crash when she was a teenager and her father, who she was not close to, subsequently fell into alcoholism and died from liver cirrhosis. As her Alzheimer's progresses, we see Alice looking at old pictures and retreating into memories of her mother and sister. Significantly, Alice is found to have a familial type of Alzheimer's which, for carriers, holds a one hundred percent chance of developing into the condition. This raises the question of whether her children – who have a fifty percent chance of carrying the gene – want to get tested themselves. *Still Alice* is a film heavily focused on the nuclear unit whereby, as Andrea Capstick (2022, personal communication, 10 October) puts it, 'the genetic chain holds the nuclear links together'.

The familial core are Alice and John Howland, a white, middle-aged couple, both very successful in their chosen fields – she a tenured university professor of linguistics at Columbia University, a private Ivy League college, and he a medical physician. They live in a large New York house and have three adult children all living away from home, and all of whom they have been able to financially support (through medical school, law school and with trying to establish an acting career). Prior to Alice's Alzheimer's diagnosis the couple were in good health, regularly jogging, travelling and enjoying social activities. The struggles encountered in the film relate to the family's grapple with Alice's declining health and its impact on familial relationships, which are undoubtedly dynamics to negotiate for anyone experiencing a diagnosis. Barriers to accessing services are not a feature of this film since the Howlands presumably have expendable income and access to high-quality, high-cost health care through insurance plans provided by their jobs.

Heterosexuality itself glides *almost* seamlessly through the film with two exceptions. There is one explicit mention of a gay roommate (who we never see) which appears to be given as a reason for establishing that he is not a potential romantic interest for the couple's younger daughter Lydia, and one allusion to homosexuality when Lydia and Alice are discussing the 1991 play *Angels in America*.[4] Lydia asks Alice 'you must've known somebody that died from AIDS, right?' and Alice replies 'Oh, yeah, honey, everybody did. We lost a lot of people'. Only two fleeting scenes, these instances may nonetheless serve to stand as the 'other' against which heterosexuality in the film can be juxtaposed as regular and taken-for-granted. Equally, in relation to the latter example, an argument can be made about the drawing of parallels between losses experienced at the height of the 1980s AIDS crisis in the US, and the loss being experienced by Alice and her family as her Alzheimer's progresses. Both AIDS and Alzheimer's have been cast by mainstream discourse as frightening, threatening pandemics and, in both cases, significant levels of stigma are experienced in relation to a diagnosis, something Glatzer and Westmoreland (the film's writers and directors) would have been all too aware of.

Over the course of the film we learn that all of the primary characters – the nuclear family members – are *doing* some kind of heterosexuality. Heterosexuality is asserted and reasserted including at points where it feels irrelevant to the plot. Alice and John, married hub of the unit, are seemingly devoted to each other and still very much in love after nearly thirty years of marriage; kisses, embraces, romantic walks on the beach, seemingly happy family meals, and playful reminiscing about the life they have had together all suggest this. Their older daughter, Anna, is married and enjoying a successful career. Early on we find out that Anna and her husband Charlie have been having trouble conceiving and are embarking on a fertility journey with the help of a private clinic. Lydia, the slightly maverick, alternative daughter who is pursuing an acting career against the wishes of her parents – Alice in particular – lives three thousand miles away in California. Around half way through the film during a lunch with Alice, Alice asks Lydia if she is involved with either one of her two male room-mates, to which she replies: 'Doug's gay. And Malcolm and I did have a thing but it's over'. This scene seems irrelevant to the overarching plot, serving little purpose other than to perhaps reassure the viewer that Lydia dates men? To communicate that Lydia is not in a stable relationship tying her to California? (a point which is seems relevant later in the story). In relation to Alice and John's son Tom, reference is made – in the opening scene - to a girlfriend he has broken up with. In a later scene Tom brings a new girlfriend, Jenny, to a thanksgiving dinner at the family home. This feels more thoughtfully integrated since it is used as a device in the film to illustrate Alice's trouble with short term memory as, although Tom introduces her to Jenny when they arrive, by the time it comes to sitting down at the table to eat Alice seems to have forgotten that they ever met and introduces herself again ('Hi, I'm Alice, lovely to meet you').

Once all of the characters have been mapped out in relation to heterosexuality, their performance of that, and other norms, is sometimes problematised in the film by other characters, implying that it is not being done properly. For example, in the opening scene of the film, Tom is late to join Alice's fiftieth birthday celebration – a nuclear family meal in an upscale restaurant. When he arrives alone Alice asks 'oh hey, isn't uh, Lisa [Tom's girlfriend] coming?' to which he replies 'no, we split up'. At this point Lydia comments, in a snide tone, 'Yes, I did notice that your status popped up as single, *yet again*', implying that he has had a tedious string of (failed) relationships. There is a reprieve for Tom though, because he is still in medical school and one heteronormative *line drawn in advance* (Ahmed, 2006) is focused on setting up a career first, particularly for men, before 'settling down' into marriage. One wonders if ideas about a 'successful' work/career life are tied up with the successful performance of family. At the same family meal, Anna asks Alice if she has spoken to Lydia. Alice says that Lydia was unable to come to the meal because she had a 'really important audition' and Anna's husband suggests this could be Lydia's big break, to which Alice replies a hesitant 'yeah, maybe' before Anna snarls 'don't hold your breath'. It is therefore established early on that Lydia is living somewhat off-script – not following a 'line drawn in advance' – which seems to cause an air of discomfort for the rest of the family.

Gender, gendered norms and expectations pertaining to gender are relevant to a consideration of the film, particularly in relation to Lydia who ends up taking on the role of primary carer for her mother, in what I read as a sort of turn to salvation. Following her diagnosis, Alice goes into a rapid decline and experiences significant deterioration in her short-term memory very quickly. At the same time her husband, John, is offered an attractive job at Mayo Clinic in Minnesota, over 2000 miles away from New York. Sympathetically portrayed as unable to cope with his wife's condition and unable (or unwilling?) to miss out on this career opportunity, John takes the job which the couple's three children appear to be supportive of ('that's great, it's absolutely the right decision' – Anna), and eventually moves to Minnesota. Given expectations related to the caregiving role and who is expected to undertake this, we – the audience – must wonder how the film would portray a wife who moved out of the family home to pursue a career instead of remaining with and caring for an unwell husband. We see virtually nothing of an emotional struggle associated with making this decision other than a brief scene when Lydia moves home to be with Alice and John says to her 'you're a better man than I am' before he breaks down crying, perhaps revealing his own sense of failure and fragile masculinity.

In the midst of Alice's advancing Alzheimer's disease, John is somehow absolved of the marriage vows ('in good health or bad') around which heteronormative expectations are often so heavily hung. The nuclear family core (Alice and John's marriage) is, ultimately, unable to withstand the difficulties it experiences as Alice's condition progresses. It is at this point in my argument that the significance of the relationship between heteronormativity and dementia may have most purchase. The implication in – or at best a point for consideration raised by – *Still Alice* is that the further progressed dementia comes for someone, the further away from the 'norm' they become; there is a point at which they inherently become too 'other' (or too queer?) to remain part of the heteronormative order of things. Alice's dementia precludes 'successful aging' – her husband seems to give up on her, prioritising his career path – and she becomes implicitly framed as a problem that needs to be dealt with and managed. We see her physical and cognitive decline, she slumps in the corner, unable to speak, whilst her family ruminates within her earshot about what can be done.

Indeed, after John has accepts the post in Minnesota, we are shown a conversation between him, Tom and Anna – them in the background of the shot whilst Alice sits in the foreground, facing away from the camera, head slumped to one side – about who will take care of Alice when John moves to Minnesota. John acknowledges neither of them would be in a position to do this: 'Now, Anna, you have the babies and you wanna go back to work, and you're not in a position to care for her, not seriously Tom, and I can't keep the Mayo waiting, at the beginning of the month I am gone. Now I want to take her with me, I will get her the best possible care'. Interestingly John lays out the reasons that his eldest daughter is unable to take on the task of caring, but needs no such reasoning for Tom's inability to do this. And although he claims to want to take Alice with him, in the end he does not do this. During an appointment with Alice's neurologist it was clear that John was well informed about Alzheimer's so he surely would have known that consistency and familiarity is particularly important for someone living with dementia meaning that relocating to a town with no familiarity or network would be detrimental. When he initially introduces the idea of taking the job, not taking it does not seem to be an option, with the implication that the family's financial life depended on it – but his current post is not under threat and, presumably, a qualified, established physician would not have trouble finding work in or near New York City.

In order for John to take up his new role, the family must find a way to make sure Alice is cared for. Anna is unable to get involved with this as she is focused on her successful family life – established career, new babies, reproducing the heteronormative nuclear family unit. At the outset of the film we learn that Alice is going through the early stages of menopause, as she tells her neurologist she initially thought the symptoms she was experiencing might be related to this. Now that she is expendable in terms of the reproductive role women are expected to take up in the family, Anna takes up the mantel. Meanwhile, whilst Tom is busy with medical school, Lydia – with no significant romantic relationship we know of, and an acting career that has yet to launch – is conveniently available. She sacrifices the pursuit of her West-Coast acting career and moves three thousand miles back to the family home so that she can live with Alice while John is working at the Mayo. This is portrayed as an opportunity for her to heal the rifts in her relationship with her mom, and to make up for the time she was far away and not around to help ('If she cared, she wouldn't be on the other side of the country' – Anna).

Interestingly, earlier in the film Lydia is set-up as occupying a care-giving role of sorts in relation to her male roommates. When Alice visits Lydia's flat she explains the mess saying that 'the boys are total slobs. The kitchen is the main battleground but I've got 'em in training so we'll see how that goes'. Once Lydia moves home, she shares caring for her mother with Elena who is a regular paid care-giver, although hardly appears in the film at all. Drawing on the elastic definitions of heteronormativity set out earlier, it is evident that gendered roles play a significant role in shoring up norms related to family life. Lydia steps in to provide the caring role which is at once afforded low social status and also – in this case – holds redeeming potential. One way or another, the film seems to be saying Lydia is doing 'the right thing' by her family and, by implication, the social order of things. There is further exploration to be undertaken in relation to the character of Elena and the significance of her role in terms of what the film is (or is not) saying about class, race and gender.

Towards the end of the film, before moving home to be with Alice, Lydia has a role in a theatre performance of Chekhov's *Three Sisters* (1901) playing Irina.[5] John, Lydia and Charlie attend and we see Lydia perform part of one of the scenes. The selection here in terms of which piece of dialogue to show Lydia delivering seems significant:

> There will come a time when everybody will know why, for what purpose, there is all this suffering, and there will be no more mysteries. But now we must live, we must work, just work! Tomorrow, I'll go away alone, and I'll teach and give my whole life to those who may perhaps, need it. It's autumn now, soon it will be winter, the snow will cover everything, and I shall be working, just working ....

This left me wondering about the potential metaphors being drawn by the films' script-writers. Is Lydia asking about the suffering experienced by her mother? Is she saying that, despite her mother's condition, they must all carry on living as much as they can? And is the work the work of finding a better way to live? Working at her relationship with her mom while she has the chance? Finding a cure for the condition? Or is it, perhaps, her own work to support her family which manifests later in the form of her moving home to be with her mother? Is the snow that covers everything the progression of the Alzheimer's disease which, it is implied, will eventually bury all of her mother's memories just as the snow will eventually cover everything?

Alice's struggle with her condition and declining memory runs in parallel with Anna's attempt to get pregnant through a fertility clinic, also a struggle of sorts. There is a juxtaposition between the downward trajectory of Alice's memory and the hope and excitement of Anna's pregnancy, announced partway through the film, and arrival of twin babies (one of whom is named Alice) near the end of the film when Alice is becoming more noticeably affected by her condition. Alice gives a keynote speech at a conference about Alzheimer's disease from the perspective of someone living with the condition. As Alice delivers the speech, focused on the concept of loss and what Alice feels she is losing, shots of her are punctuated with shots of Anna who is in the audience holding her pregnant belly. Alice tells her audience she is not suffering but 'struggling to be a part of things, to stay connected to whom I once was'. Whilst Alice's life moves further away from the 'normal' that she knows and is invested in, Anna is cementing her own nuclear unit with (biological) children, one of the ultimate lynchpins of 'normal' family life. Of what it is like to live with Alzheimer's, Alice says 'on my good days, I can [...] almost pass for a normal person'. This is a telling comment which reveals the power of wanting to be, or trying to be, 'normal', a struggle quietly expressed and troubled, throughout the film.

Conclusion

The Howland family epitomises the kind of 'normal' family life that the lens of heteronormativity seeks to describe and unsettle in terms of societal expectations and pressures. This family represents the 'normal' core that these expectations supposedly work for, and on an initial viewing it would be easy to read the film – as I did – as simply perpetuating normative ideas about intimate and family life: the depiction of a privileged family, the assertion and reassertion of heterosexuality, However, a closer reading over several more viewings allowed me to develop a more nuanced analysis as the fragility of normative heterosexuality in the film became apparent, which unsettled its normalised status.

I hope to have shown how a close reading of film drawing on the analytical lens of heteronormativity can be fruitful for critical dementia studies, laying the groundwork for further work of this kind. I located the concept theoretically and, based on my earlier work in this area, I outlined some elastic features related to heteronormativity, providing a framework for reading film – or any other text – through this critical lens. A reading through the critical lens of heteronormativity was applied to the film *Still Alice* to explore how it might be operationalised and applied in practice. In the course of applying the framework in my reading of this film, I developed my original framework, adding two additional points for consideration. The framework should remain elastic and open to modification based on its application in relation to cultural texts or data.

Ryan and Lenos (2020) point out that all films contain historical, political, cultural, psychological, social and economic meanings, referring to the cultural-context they were made in a multitude of ways (for a parallel discussion of the representation of dementia in life writing, see Hartung's discussion of Liv Ullmann's *Die Urolige* in Chapter 5). The argument set forward here is that *Still Alice* reflects the cultural context out of which it emerges, at once perpetuating and unsettling normative expectations about family life, particularly in relation to how dementia is read and represented. Of particular significance is the argument about the way in which Alice is othered as a result of her dementia as this disrupts the heteronormative order of family life, particularly in relation to the healthy body and mind. This raises the question about the extent to which people living with dementia might be held/positioned in a kind of (queer) juxtaposition as a troubling 'other' against which the set of norms around which family life is so often hung relies.

Notes

1 Heteronormativity has also frequently been used in this way outside of the dementia field.
2 Iris (2001); The Notebook (2004); Away From Her (2006).
3 See, for example, Foucault (1976) on theorising categories of sexuality as socially constructed; hooks (1981), Lorde (1983) and Anzaldua (1981) on the importance of interrogating the complexities of identity and difference); and Rich (1980), Rubin (1975) and Wittig (1981) on the exposition of heterosexuality as a powerful social institution.
4 A two-part play by Tony Kushner which examines AIDS and homosexuality in 1980s North America.
5 There are some notable parallels between the characters of Irina and Lydia; both are youngest sisters; both leave home to explore work ambitions; both experience pain/loss and immediately thereafter throw themselves into gender approved roles (Irina teaching, Lydia 'caring').

References

Ahmed, S. (2004). *The Cultural Politics of Emotion*. Edinburgh: Edinburgh University Press.

Ahmed, S. (2006). *Queer Phenomenology*. Durham: Duke University Press.

Away From Her. 2006. [Film]. Sarah Polly. dir. Scotland: Foundry Films.

Behuniak, S.M. (2010). The living dead? The construction of people with Alzheimer's disease as zombies. *Ageing and Society*, 31 (1): 70–92. https://doi.org/10.1017/S0144686X10000693

Berlant, L. and Warner, M. (2000). Sex in public. In Berlant, L. (ed.), *Intimacy*. Chicago: University of Chicago Press, 311–330.

Capstick, A., Chatwin, J. and Ludwin, K. (2014). Challenging representations of debehmentia in contemporary Western fiction film: from epistemic injustice to social participation. In Swinner, J. and Schweda, M. (eds.), *Popularizing Dementia – Public Expressions and Representations of Forgetfulness*. Aging Studies Thematic Volume VI. Transcript Verlag: Bielefeld, 7–29.

Chambers, S.A. (2007). 'An Incalculable Effect': Subversions of Heteronormativity. *Political Studies*, 55 (3), 656–679. https://doi.org/10.1111/j.1467-9248.2007.00654.x

Chekhov, A. (1901). *Three Sisters*. Adolf Marks: St. Petersburg.

Davis, L.J. (2006). Constructing normalcy: The bell curve, the novel, and the invention of the disabled body in the nineteenth century. In Davis, L.J. (ed.), *The Disability Studies Reader*. 2nd ed. New York: Routledge, 3–20.

Di Lorito, C. Bosco, A. Peel, E. Hinchliff, S. Dening, T. Calasanti, T. de Vries, B. Cutler, N. Fredriksen-Goldsen, K.I. and Harwood, R.H. (2021). Are dementia services and support organisations meeting the needs of Lesbian, Gay, Bisexual and Transgender (LGBT) caregivers of LGBT people living with dementia? A scoping review of the literature. *Aging & Mental Health*, 26 (10). https://doi.org/10.1080/13607863.2021.2008870

Edelman, L. (2004). *No Future: Queer Theory and the Death Drive*. Duke University Press: Durham

Falcus, S. (2014). Storying Alzheimer's Disease in Lisa Genova's Still Alice. Entertext, 11. ISSN 14723085.

Foucault, M. (1979) [1976]. *The History of Sexuality Volume 1: An Introduction.* London: Allen Lane. ISBN 978-0-7139-1094-0.

Genova, L (2007). *Still Alice.* London: Pocket Books.

Herz, M. and Johansson, T. (2015). The normativity of the concept of heteronormativity. *Journal of Homosexuality*, 62(8), 1009–1020.

hooks, b. (1981). *Ain't I a Woman? Black Women and Feminism.* Boston: South End Press.

Iris. (2001). [Film]. Richard Eyre. dir. USA: Miramax.

Jackson, S. (1999). *Heterosexuality in Question.* London: SAGE.

Jackson, S. (2006a). Gender, sexuality and heterosexuality: The complexity (and limits) of heteronormativity. *Feminist Theory*, 7 (1), 105–121.

Jutel, A. G. (2019). *Diagnosis.* Toronto: University of Toronto Press.

King, A. (2021). Queer futures? Forget it! Dementia, queer theory and the limits of normativity. *Journal of Aging Studies*, 63. doi:10.1016/j.jaging.2021.100993.

Lorde, A. (1983). *Zami: A New Spelling of My Name.* Freedom: The Crossing Press.

Ludwin, K. (2011). 'Negotiating normative heterosexuality: A biographical-narrative study in the New Town of Milton Keynes'. PhD. Birkbeck College, University of London. London.

Ludwin, K. (2016). 'Heteronormativity and dementia: What's the relevance?', 27th April 2016. Available at: http://blogs.brad.ac.uk/dementia/heteronormativity-and-dementia-whats-the-relevance/ (Accessed 27th April 2016).

Marchia, J. and Sommer, J.M. (2019). (Re)defining heteronormativity. *Sexualities*, 22 (3). https://doi.org/10.1177/1363460717741801

Mikos, L. (2014). Analysis of Film. In Flick, U. (ed.). *The SAGE Handbook of Qualitative Data Analysis.* London: SAGE, 394–408.

Peel, E. and McDaid, S. (2015). *'Over the Rainbow' Lesbian, Gay, Bisexual and Trans People and Dementia Project Summary Report.* Dementia Engagement and Empowerment Project.

Price, E. (2012). Gay and lesbian carers: Ageing in the shadow of dementia. *Ageing and Society*, 32(3): 516–532.

Rich, A. (1980). Compulsory heterosexuality and lesbian existence. In Abelove, H. Aina Barale, M., and Halperin, D.M. (eds.), 1993. *The Lesbian and Gay Studies Reader.* London: Routledge, 227–254.

Richardson, D. (1996), ed. *Theorising Heterosexualiity.* Buckingham: Open University Press.

Rosenfeld, D. (2009). Heteronormativity and homonormativity as practical and moral resources: The case of lesbian and gay elders. *Gender & Society*, 23 (5): 617–638.

Rubin, G. (1975). The traffic in women: Notes on the 'political economy' of sex. In: Reiter, R., ed. *Toward an Anthropology of Women.* New York: Monthly Review Press, 157–210.

Ryan, M. and Lenos, M. (2020). *An Introduction to Film Analysis: Technique and Meaning in Narrative Film.* Bloomsbury

Sandberg, L. J. and Marshall, B.L. (2017). Queering aging futures. *Societies*, 7(21): 1–11.

Stasińska, Agata (2018), *Socjologia pary: praktyki intymne w związkach nieheteroseksualnych.* Kraków: Nomos.

Still Alice. (2014). [Film]. Richard Glatzer and Wash Westmoreland. dirs. USA: Lutzus-Brown.

Supernova. (2020). [Film]. Harry Macqueen. dir. UK: The Bureau.

Szlendak, Tomasz (2015). Socjologia rodziny: ewolucja, historia, zróżnicowanie, Warszawa, PWN.

The Notebook. (2004). [Film]. Nick Cassavetes. dir. USA: New Line Cinema.

Ward, R. and Price, E. (2016). Reconceptualising dementia: Towards a politics of senility. In Westwood, S. and Price, E. (eds.), *Lesbian, Gay, Bisexual and Trans* Individuals Living with Dementia.* London: Routledge, 85–98.

Warner, M. (1991). Fear of a queer planet. *Social Text*, 29 (3): 3–17.

West, C. and Zimmerman, D.J. (1987). Doing gender. *Gender and Society*, 1 (2): 125–121.

Williams, F. (2004). *Rethinking Families.* London: Calouste Gulbenkian Foundation.

Wittig, M. (1981). One is not born a woman. In. Wittig, M., 1992, *The Straight Mind.* Boston: Beacon Press, 9–21.

Yuval-Davis, N. (1993). The (dis)comfort of being 'hetero'. In Wilkinson, S. and Kitzinger, C. (eds.), *Heterosexuality.* London: SAGE, 52–53.

8 Race, ethnicity and culture

Problematic application in dementia and old age

*Moïse Roche, Maria Zubair,
and James Rupert Fletcher*

Introduction: Ethnogerontological imperatives

Since 2020, racial and ethnic inequalities in COVID-19 mortality and morbidity have once again concentrated attention on the role of race and ethnicity in the field of health and ageing (Bhala et al., 2020). From the outset of the pandemic, predictions of the most dooming impact on Black African countries occupied international news, with various sources projecting the deadliest outcomes in Black African communities; later having to make circumspect retractions (Soy, 2020; Witchalls, 2021). Although these predictions did not eventuate into the devastating consequences seen in Black and South Asian communities in the USA and the UK, inequalities in populations the most affected by the COVID-19 pandemic have added renewed urgency to the sense that lessons need to be learned from issues of racial, ethnic or cultural differences in health and illness (Ayanian & Buntin, 2020).

Besides the new threat of COVID-19, population ageing in the UK, as in other developed countries, has also revitalised academic and professional interest in ethnogerontology. England, for example, has a racially and ethnically diverse population, which is gradually increasing in size and age. Since the 1991 census, the population described as Black and Minority Ethnic (BME[1]) has risen from 3 to 7 million in 2011, with the African community one of the largest areas of growth (Jivraj, 2012). Whilst BME communities have in general younger population structures than those of the White population (Moriarty et al., 2011), there has been a steady increase in the number of Black African and Caribbean older people as the first generation of migrants who moved to the UK during the 1950s age. By 2051, the highest proportion of people aged 50 and over is projected to be of BME descent (Wohland et al., 2010). Given that the incidence of dementia rises with age, the rapid ageing of this population means that the number of BME people with dementia will also grow rapidly (Knapp et al., 2007; Prince et al., 2014).

Amid contemporary ethnogerontological imperatives, there has been a recent increase in calls for action, investment and research to reduce racial and ethnic health inequality in dementia and later life. Dementia may be as old as mankind itself (Boller & Forbes, 1998), with origins of its concept traced as far back as the year 2000 BC (Signoret & Hauw, 1991), but its association with race, ethnicity or culture is relatively recent. The body of literature on the history of dementia does

DOI: 10.4324/9781003290353-12

not make references to early interconnection between dementia, race and/or ethnicity, nor does it mention when this relationship first began (Boller, 2008; Boller & Forbes, 1998; Signoret & Hauw, 1991). (In Chapter 2, Capstick critiques this inattentiveness to the effects of major 20th century histories, such as mass migration, on the lives of contemporary people with dementia). In our previous work, we noted a rapid increase, in recent decades, in publications especially during the 21st century that focused their analysis on the relationship between race, ethnicity and culture, and dementia (Fletcher et al., 2021).

Beyond publications, race and ethnicity have entered into the wider dementia research economy. Through the 2010s, Alzheimer's Society UK developed a dedicated 'BAME'[1] portfolio comprised of several research projects, supported with funding of around £2.4 million (Alzheimer's Society UK, 2022) (Fletcher discusses the wider financial development of a dementia economy in Chapter 1). Over recent years, notable organisations, such as Alzheimer's Society Canada, have released statements not only condemning racism in response to the Black Lives Matter movement but also promising to change the way they attend to race, ethnicity and dementia in their localities (Alzheimer Society Canada, 2021). In 2021, the Alzheimer's Association released a report dedicated to examining 'Racial and Ethnic Attitudes on Alzheimer's and Dementia Care' (Alzheimer's Association, 2021). The organisation also emphasised racial health inequalities when contesting regulation of the Alzheimer's drug aducanumab (Azheimer's Association, 2022) by the Centers for Medicare & Medicaid Services. Hence, race and ethnicity have latterly come to feature more centrally in the dementia research economy in various ways (part of a wider attentiveness to intersectionalities discussed by Lotherington in Chapter 6).

This apparent recent interest in race, ethnicity and culture in dementia research seems to coincide with a growth in literature about dementia awareness (Fletcher, 2020). The positioning of race/ethnicity in dementia awareness research as deficient resembles the history of various psychiatric disorders and the media landscape that have embraced and perpetuated the trope of the 'uneducated primitive' Black individual in need of basic education to recognise when s/he is unwell. The framing of mental health in Black communities has a long history in Eurocentric writings (Lipsedge & Littlewood, 2005) that have galvanised debates about their inherent and persistent form of racism, devaluation and dehumanisation of certain racial and ethnic groups (Fernando, 2010). For there is a clear sense of implicit racism in mostly White disciplines vilifying an exclusively Black group (Bhambra, 2017; Boyd et al., 2020; Rai et al., 2022; Sims-Schouten & Gilbert, 2022).

A hot-off-the-press UK Dementia Research Institute report urges the British Government to prioritise funding for scientific innovation, to facilitate larger inclusive dementia trials and develop effective strategies to address racial and ethnic dementia inequalities (UKDRI, 2022). This heightened attentiveness to the interconnections between race, ethnicity and dementia has also brought an acceleration of publications highlighting prevailing racial and ethnic inequalities in dementia rates, diagnosis, outcomes and service access (Fitzpatrick et al., 2004; Katz et al., 2012; Knapp et al., 2007; Mehta & Yeo, 2017; Prince et al., 2014). Much of the resulting work has remained ensconced in the deliberation of racial/ethnic differences and distinctions. As such, minoritised ethnic groups have borne the brunt of practices of categorising medical meanings in relation to race and ethnicity. That dementia is racialised – and/or ethnicised – and problematised in some ethnicities and not others is the theme of this chapter, as is the need to separate out the different meanings of race and ethnicity and understand how they relate to health, ageing and dementia. Below, we expand on our previous arguments regarding the ethnicity problem of dementia (Fletcher et al., 2021) and make a number of additional observations. Notably, we argue that to better understand the place of race and/or ethnicity in dementia studies, a broader historical and social perspective is needed. We also examine and consider the concepts of race, ethnicity and culture, and discuss their meaning and significance in relation to identity, health, ageing and dementia. We posit that defaulting to race, ethnicity and culture as intrinsic risk factors for dementia among minoritised older people with dementia, the people researchers set out to give voice to, might instead compound a sense of disempowerment and risk misrepresenting these groups and their interests. That said, our analysis can apply to other conditions and areas of research given the process of racialisation is not specific or restrictive to dementia and ageing. Race, ethnicity and culture: meaning and problematic application.

As in all enquiries about race and ethnicity, this chapter relies on (and unavoidably perpetuates) the definitions and classifications of population grouping. The terms and language used to describe and report on different racial, ethnic and cultural groups vary substantially around the world, with no clear consensus on preferred and acceptable terminology. There are inherent difficulties and ethical complexities in writing about such concepts as race, ethnicity and culture as they are dynamic, unscientific, contentious and often contested. As identification grounds, they are rooted in social interactions, draw heavily on commonplace assumptions, general narrative, popular usage and the social zeitgeist as well as historical and political context. Despite these difficulties, they are regarded as readily and socially understandable to a point that allows the drawing of lines of separation between racial and ethnic group members and non-members.

In the interest of clarity, we decided to adopt minoritised ethnic in this chapter to describe any specific group of people who, by virtue of numerical size and in relation to current conventions of race, ethnicity and place of residence, is in a minority. We use 'minoritised' instead of 'minority' from a social constructionist standpoint to show that minoritisation is a social process that places people into minority status based on circumstances rather than their intrinsic and inherent characteristics (Gunaratnam, 2003; Predelli et al., 2012). We recognise that the term minoritised ethnic is used in many ways and is location sensitive, and that everyone can belong to a minoritised ethnicity depending on where they live.

It is important to elucidate, even briefly, the constructs of race, ethnicity and culture given they are used routinely in dementia research and practice, as in other settings, without a clear understanding of their immediate and underlying meanings. Distinguishing race, ethnicity and culture is also necessary as these constructs are too often conflated and treated as interchangeable in making sense of health disparities. Not making this distinction runs the risk of overlooking critical determinants of racial inequalities in health such as racism and racialisation, as well as failing to understand the pathways through which race and ethnicity affect health and dementia outcomes (Barot & Bird, 2001; Miles, 2004; Neblett Jr, 2019).

Races have often been distinguished on the basis of vague phenotypic characteristics, especially skin colour, facial structure, hair type and colour, and eye colour (Dennis, 1995). Whereas ethnic distinctions have tended to focus on even more unclear and difficult to determine cultural characteristics such as history, language, religion, and closeness in physical characteristics (Montagu, 1942). As for culture, designated as an important dimension of ethnicity, it is equally elusive in that it relates to shared and learned values, behaviours, beliefs and attitudes that are purported to make people behave in a certain way (Corin, 1995). With much evolution in the definitions and applications of these constructs, which are, in themselves, dynamic, heterogeneous, subjective, often self-classified and presumed, there is no universally accepted definition for race and ethnicity. This makes ethnicity-focused dementia studies a challenge when we attempt to understand to whom they apply (Roche et al., 2021).

The notion of classifying people by race based on observation of physical similarities and differences originates from 18th-century naturalists and philosopher (Smedley et al., 2017) and is grounded in highly discredited early 19th/20th-century racist scientific studies that used comparison of the physiognomy of Black and White individuals to divide populations (Gould & Gold, 1996; Guthrie, 2004; Washington, 2006; Williams, 1997). These racial divisions were conferred an aura of scientific credibility in writings by people with vested interests in maintaining distinction and separation of people to retain and optimise personal financial gain and legitimise horrific biomedical experimentation in the name of scientific advancements, on the people they had dehumanised (Fernando, 2010).

Using race, ethnicity and culture as variables in dementia research is challenging and highly problematic, not only because of their ambiguous and contentious definitions but also because of their prejudicial nature and socio-political implications (Lin & Kelsey, 2000). Even though these constructs have no objective or externally valid scientific basis, and rely heavily on commonplace assumptions and general sense to obtain meanings, they are often used in the framing and interpretation of research, and promptly transformed into risk factors for ill health (but, notably, not good health). Despite these difficulties, race and ethnicity are rarely challenged or opened to scrutiny in dementia research.

Identification grounds, biological proxies and cultural essentialism

Race and ethnicity are identification grounds on which assumptions are made about certain people based on constellations of characteristics (Jenkins, 2008, 2014). When applied, these form crude categorisations treated as deterministic of who people are and predictive of how they behave (Cornell & Hartmann, 2006). Race and social scholars have long debunked essentialist understandings of race and ethnicity, and have moved towards more socially nuanced perspectives on these identification grounds as processes rooted in social and historic contexts (Jenkins, 1997). Nevertheless, essentialising assumptions are commonplace in health and medical scholarships that generate and articulate race/ethnicity-associated 'problems' and related knowledges (Torres, 2019).

Dementia research is not exempt from these difficulties. Some scholars focus their analyses of minoritised populations through lenses of race and ethnicity as biological explanations for observed racial and ethnic disparities. In the UK, Dementia Research Institute report mentioned earlier, leading dementia scientists are described as having convened to better understand 'the genetic role of ethnicity in determining dementia risk' (UKDRI, 2022). Such articulation of dementia in relation to ethnicity unwittingly problematises minoritised ethnicities as deficient by virtue of their ethnically intrinsic make-up, and in comparison with a flawed notion of a homogeneous 'White group', presented as the default category with regard to which the dementia outcomes and experiences of minoritised races and ethnicities are made sense of.

It has now been well-established that race and ethnicity cannot be used as proxies for biology (Foster & Sharp, 2002), as they lack consistency in their genetic composition and display greater (intragroup) genetic variation among individuals within the same racial categories than between individuals of different racial categories (intergroup)(Cooper, 2003; Senior & Bhopal, 1994; Tishkoff & Kidd, 2004; Williams et al., 1994). As such the biological conception of race has received strong oppositions and been marked as 'non-existent' in scientific terms (Beutler et al., 1996; Bradby, 1995; Chaturvedi & McKeigue, 1994; McKenney & Bennett, 1994; Senior & Bhopal, 1994; Williams et al., 1994), given that genetic differences between humans are 'inconsistent and typically insignificant' (Cashmore, 2004; Cornell & Hartmann, 2006). There are no genetic variants that occur in a racial group that cannot be found in another. There is, however, a risk that overemphasising racial predispositions for disease, even when genetic evidence is lacking, may catalyse researchers' biases, exacerbating prejudice towards marginalised racial and/or ethnic groups (Cooper, 2003).

Scholars and other stakeholders involved in dementia research and practice need to reflect on their engagements with race and ethnicity, not only in how they use these constructs but how they articulate study findings and the conclusions that are drawn from their observations based on apparent racial and ethnic differences (Fletcher et al., 2021). The ways in which scientific communities conceptualise the relationship between racial and ethnic categories and genetic variation can be problematic in that they fabricate risks for all members of those categories and create damaging narratives that influence lay perceptions of the nature of racial and ethnic groups. As it is not possible to determine the location of the boundaries of racial and ethnic groups biologically, it behoves scientific communities to pay attention to the social constitution of populations and corresponding mechanisms through which race and ethnicity relate to health disparities.

That said, one cannot simply escape these problems by attending to the social delineation of groups as a substitute for biological approaches. The development of dementia studies scholarship regarding ethnicity throughout the 21st century has often attended to cultural meanings to make sense of the assumed difference of minoritised groups, fully recognising that said groups are not coherent biological categories. However, in practice, culture can be weaponised in much the same manner, implying that there is some essential (cultural) characteristic of particular groups that impacts upon dementia, typically in a negative manner. This is evident in claims that a particular group does not 'properly' engage with dementia and therefore suffers negative outcomes. For example, multiple studies have associated South Asian culture with stigma of mental illness and dementia, as well as designating their apparent reluctance to engage with services for these conditions as culturally rooted (Giebel et al., 2015; Mukadam et al., 2015; Seabrooke et al., 2004; Werner et al., 2012). (This can be based around uses of language, as discussed by Koncul, and colleagues in Chapter 4). Moreover, the proper-ness of said engagement and the negative-ness of the outcomes is typically defined by majority ethnic researchers (Fletcher, 2020; Fletcher et al., 2021). Ultimately, while many dementia studies scholars may reject the biological essentialism of ethnicity-related research, culturally essentialist approaches can be similarly problematic.

The culture-centred approach to race and ethnicity can become a means through which minoritised people affected by dementia can be made responsible by well-intentioned but conceptually naïve dementia scholarship. Exposed to the quadruple jeopardy of dementia, covid (Godfrey et al., 2021), race and ageing (Chatters et al., 2020), rapidly ageing minoritised ethnic communities are often repeatedly presented as being somewhat responsible for their apparent susceptibility to diseases. This implicitly attributes blame – if not on biological basis, then on cultural basis – and demarcates these communities as the focus of increased attention in race/ethnicity-focused dementia research (Fox & Petersen, 2013), which is not always to the benefit of these communities.

The dangers of situating the consequences of race and ethnicity with individuals or groups in reference to 'culture' have been illustrated in recent history by the cultural deficiency model, which is now 'abandoned' and highly criticised (Moore, 2008; Salkind, 2008). The model asserts that minoritised group members are different because their culture is dysfunctional and lacking important characteristics. By drawing attention to racial and ethnic disparities and presenting one side as deficient in comparison to another, the model homogenises and pathologises the group's cultural values and inculpates families with transmitting the pathology (Harry & Klingner, 2007; Kirk & Goon, 1975; Solorzano, 1992). In response to criticism of this model, the term of 'cultural deficiency' is now rarely used. However, the underlying perspective and associated beliefs of the cultural deficiency model still permeate society and dementia studies. It continues to influence research, psychological theories and even political views under more recently popularised and adopted terms such as 'cultural diversity' and 'cultural difference'. In her work on situating dementia prevention, Leibing (2018) notes that if some people are more affected by an illness because they face adverse social circumstances, there is an irony in society positioning the responsibility for reducing that risk at the level of the individual and their essentialised cultural characteristics, conceived as though somehow isolated from society more broadly.

Ultimately, culture runs into similar problems to those that undermine biological (mis)conceptions. As research around the differential impact of dementia and the coronavirus (COVID-19) have shown, generic and collective categories such as Black Caribbean, Indian, White British and Pakistani are problematic as they offer little clarity on the identity of the people they purport to describe (Bhala et al., 2020). This is further exacerbated by the use of broad cumbersome descriptors such as BME and BAME (Black, Asian and Minority Ethnic) that aggregate multiple groups of people. These terms, which are widely used in UK, were arguably introduced to address the complexities of a multicultural society. They have instead perpetuated a culture of racial dichotomy of 'Whiteness vs Otherness', a framing which was brought about by racist science that still affects minoritised ethnic groups and their participation in research (Malik, 1996; Saeed et al., 2020; Scarman, 1986).

Critical engagements with minoritisation

It is important to clarify, and indeed emphasise, that we are not arguing for the eradication of race and ethnicity as considerations in dementia studies. The categorisation of human characteristics and experiences is an essential component of health and social research. Instead, we suggest that categories need to be as meaningful as possible, acknowledge the diversity of human populations, and incorporate an alertness to both their own limitations and their generative capacities, whereby using certain categories reinforces their imposition on the real world. These caveats are vital if research findings are to be useful and relevant to the people they purport to describe. Without such caveats, the use of racial and ethnic categorisation, even in well-intentioned research, risks being useful for stakeholders in the research economy only.

We say this because there is a risk that dementia scholarship, recognising the problems of the field's recent interest in ethnicity, inadvertently erases significant aspects of the dementia experiences of minoritised ethnic groups through the use of what it may consider to be more politically correct notions to avoid uncomfortableness of dealing with racism and racial discrimination (Torres, 2020). This could explain why a rising number of scholars argue for the phasing out of racial and ethnic categories in biological sciences and health research, or at least their deconstruction into more specific indicators of health disparities between groups (Dilworth-Anderson et al., 2008; Manly, 2005, 2006). Such an approach rather misses the conceptual point at the heart of minoritisation, i.e., that there are structural inequalities by virtue of the processes of minoritisation, and those inequalities warrant our attention and action. Hence, race and ethnicity might be more useful if conceptualised as minoritising political categories through which health disparities are produced and upheld.

Beyond more nuanced conceptual schemas, there are also important questions to be asked about the practical payoff of the newfound popularity of race and ethnicity in dementia studies. A review of interventions intended to improve access to dementia services for people from minoritised ethnic groups resulted in being predominantly about educational campaigns seeking to increase awareness and re-duce stigma about dementia (Mukadam et al., 2013). Such approaches ascribe an implicit blame to minoritised people as the underlying cause of their experiences of inaccessibility, and by extension place an onus on those people to solve the problem by educating themselves. Perhaps unsurprisingly, few of these projects reported any measurable outcomes of their interventions (Mukadam et al., 2013). A culture-centred approach to ethnicity in dementia studies risks perpetuating these types of educational interventions, because they imply that the problematic aspects of dementia are rooted in shared misunderstandings among minoritised people, la-belled 'culture', rather than attending to the structural factors that place said people in circumstances more conducive to negative experiences of dementia.

While there is a newfound urgency in appeals to attend to racial and ethnic ine-qualities in relation to dementia, there is evidently a troubling lack of attentiveness to developing meaningful work and effective strategies to address these issues in a comprehensive way (Department of Health, 2015; Downs & Baj, 2015). Interest in the role of race and ethnicity in dementia has remained largely theoretical, carried out by people from majority ethnic groups and who do not have dementia. Conse-quently, much of the resulting scholarship reads more closely to engagements in intellectual exercises designed by and for an audience not directly affected by these issues than a genuine attempt to improve the circumstance of the communities most at risk of dementia. These problems have been highlighted before, but they remain unaddressed as research findings have not translated into measurable and effective actions (Blakemore & Boneham, 1994).

This begs the question of how a critical dementia studies might more fruitfully engage with minoritised experiences of dementia, with a view towards improv-ing those experiences where desirable. Importantly, what is deemed to be 'desir-able' should be defined as such by minoritised people affected by dementia and not based on the normative values or commitments of majority ethnicity researchers. Common outcome measures such as diagnosis rates and medication use should be appraised by people affected by dementia from minoritised ethnic groups, based on their preferences. Such an approach must begin from a position of respect for heterogeneity of experiences and values, and must avoid perpetuating racial and ethnic hierarchies, no matter how implicit and softly phrased in terms of 'culture' and the like. Intriguingly, these are ethical commitments that have been central to much dementia studies since the 1990s, which has pursued the meaningful inclu-sion of people with dementia. A critical dementia studies should therefore aim to continue to develop such commitments in reference to minoritised people affected by dementia.

Note

1 BME/BAME: Black (Asian) and Minority Ethnic are collective administrative terms used in UK to describe groups of people who are not identified as White British. The use of these terms has been criticised for failing to distinguish between race and ethnic-ity, for being ambiguous and lacking substantive meaning and representativeness of the people they purport to describe, while concealing some minoritised groups, notably

White minoritised groups. For a critical review of racial and ethnic terminology, see Aspinall (2020).

References

Alzheimer Society Canada. (2021). *Race and dementia* (We're changing how we see, discuss and learn about race and dementia in Canada, Issue. https://alzheimer.ca/en/take-action/change-minds/race-dementia

Alzheimer's Association. (2021). *New Alzheimer's Association Report Examines Racial and Ethnic Attitudes on Alzheimer's and Dementia Care*. https://www.alz.org/news/2021/new-alzheimers-association-report-examines-racial

Alzheimer's Society UK. (2022). *Black, Asian and minority ethnic communities and dementia research. Research – For researchers*. Retrieved 11 September 2022, from https://www.alzheimers.org.uk/for-researchers/black-asian-and-minority-ethnic-communities-and-dementia-research

Aspinall, P. J. (2020). Ethnic/racial terminology as a form of representation: A critical review of the lexicon of collective and specific terms in use in Britain. *Genealogy, 4*(3), 87.

Ayanian, J. Z., & Buntin, M. B. (2020). In pursuit of a deeper understanding of racial justice and health equity. JAMA Health Forum.

Azheimer's Association. (2022). Alzheimer's Association Statement on CMS Draft Decision. Retrieved 11 September 2022, from https://www.alz.org/news/2022/alzheimers-association-statement-on-cms-draft-deci

Barot, R., & Bird, J. (2001). Racialization: The genealogy and critique of a concept. *Ethnic and Racial Studies, 24*(4), 601–618.

Beutler, L. E., Brown, M. T., Crothers, L., Booker, K., & Seabrook, M. K. (1996). The dilemma of factitious demographic distinctions in psychological research. *Journal of Consulting and Clinical Psychology, 64*(5), 892.

Bhala, N., Curry, G., Martineau, A. R., Agyemang, C., & Bhopal, R. (2020). Sharpening the global focus on ethnicity and race in the time of COVID-19. *The Lancet, 395*(10238), 1673–1676.

Bhambra, G. K. (2017). Brexit, Trump, and 'methodological whiteness': On the misrecognition of race and class. *The British journal of sociology, 68*, S214–S232.

Blakemore, K., & Boneham, M. (1994). *Age, Race and Ethnicity: A Comparative Approach. Rethinking Ageing Series*. Bristol: Open University Press.

Boller, F. (2008). History of dementia. *Handbook of Clinical Neurology, 89*, 3–13.

Boller, F., & Forbes, M. M. (1998). History of dementia and dementia in history: An overview. *Journal of the Neurological Sciences, 158*(2), 125–133.

Boyd, R. W., Lindo, E. G., Weeks, L. D., & McLemore, M. R. (2020). On racism: A new standard for publishing on racial health inequities. *Health Affairs Blog, 10*(10.1377), 1.

Bradby, H. (1995). Ethnicity: Not a black and white issue: A research note. *Sociology of Health & Illness, 17*(3), 405–417.

Cashmore, E. (2004). *Encyclopedia of Race and Ethnic Studies*. New York: Routledge.

Chatters, L. M., Taylor, H. O., & Taylor, R. J. (2020). Older Black Americans during COVID-19: Race and age double jeopardy. *Health Education & Behavior, 47*(6), 855–860.

Chaturvedi, N., & McKeigue, P. M. (1994). Methods for epidemiological surveys of ethnic minority groups. *Journal of Epidemiology & Community Health, 48*(2), 107–111.

Cooper, R. S. (2003). Race and genomics. *The New England Journal of Medicine, 348*(12), 1166.

Corin, E. (1995). The cultural frame: Context and meaning in the construction of health. In BC Amick, S. Levine, AR Tarlov, D. Chapman Walsh (eds.) *Society and Health*. New York: Oxford University Press.

Cornell, S., & Hartmann, D. (2006). *Ethnicity and Race: Making Identities in a Changing World*. Thousand Oaks: SAGE Publications.

Dennis, R. M. (1995). Social Darwinism, scientific racism, and the metaphysics of race. *Journal of Negro Education*, 64, 243–252.

Department of Health. (2015). Prime Minister's Challenge on Dementia 2020. In: Department of Health London, UK.

Dilworth-Anderson, P., Hendrie, H. C., Manly, J. J., Khachaturian, A. S., & Fazio, S. (2008). Diagnosis and assessment of Alzheimer's disease in diverse populations. *Alzheimer's & Dementia: The Journal of the Alzheimer's Association*, 4, 305–309.

Downs, M., & Baj, N. (2015). Promoting social health for people affected by dementia: An online module for National Health Service staff. *International Psychogeriatrics*, 1, S27–S28. http://ovidsp.ovid.com/ovidweb.cgi?T=JS&CSC=Y&NEWS=N&PAGE=fulltext&D=emed16&AN=72187852

Fernando, S. (2010). *Mental Health, Race and Culture*. Basingstoke: Macmillan International Higher Education.

Fitzpatrick, A. L., Kuller, L. H., Ives, D. G., Lopez, O. L., Jagust, W., Breitner, J. C., Jones, B., Lyketsos, C., & Dulberg, C. (2004). Incidence and prevalence of dementia in the cardiovascular health study. *Journal of the American Geriatrics Society*, *52*(2), 195–204. http://ovidsp.ovid.com/ovidweb.cgi?T=JS&CSC=Y&NEWS=N&PAGE=fulltext&D=psyc4&AN=2004-10496-004

Fletcher, J. R. (2020). Positioning ethnicity in dementia awareness research: does the use of senility risk ascribing racialised knowledge deficits to minority groups? *Sociology of Health & Illness*, *42*(4), 705–723.

Fletcher, J. R., Zubair, M., & Roche, M. (2022). The neuropsychiatric biopolitics of dementia and its ethnicity problem. *The Sociological Review*, 70, 1005–1024, 00380261211059920.

Foster, M. W., & Sharp, R. R. (2002). Race, ethnicity, and genomics: Social classifications as proxies of biological heterogeneity. *Genome Research*, *12*(6), 844–850.

Fox, N. C., & Petersen, R. C. (2013). The G8 Dementia Research Summit–a starter for eight? *The Lancet*, *382*(9909), 1968.

Giebel, C. M., Zubair, M., Jolley, D., Bhui, K. S., Purandare, N., Worden, A., & Challis, D. (2015). South Asian older adults with memory impairment: Improving assessment and access to dementia care. *International Journal of Geriatric Psychiatry*, *30*(4), 345–356. Doi: 10.1002/gps.4242. http://onlinelibrary.wiley.com/doi/10.1002/gps.4242/abstract

Godfrey, W., Godfrey, W., Xu, L., Magnabosco, L., Takahashi, P., & Chandra, A. (2021). Double in jeopardy: A global pandemic-induced dyadic dementia dilemma. *Journal of the American Medical Directors Association*, *22*(3), B6.

Gould, S. J., & Gold, S. J. (1996). *The Mismeasure of Man*. New York: WW Norton & Company.

Gunaratnam, Y. (2003). *Researching 'Race' and Ethnicity: Methods, Knowledge and Power*. London: SAGE.

Guthrie, R. V. (2004). *Even the Rat was White: A Historical View of Psychology*. London: Pearson Education.

Harry, B., & Klingner, J. (2007). Discarding the deficit model. *Educational Leadership*, *64*(5), 16. https://ucl-new-primo.hosted.exlibrisgroup.com/openurl/UCL/UCL_VU2?sid=OVID:embase&id=pmid:&id=doi:10.1017%2FS1041610215002148&issn=1041-6102&isbn=&vol

ume=27&issue=SUPPL.+1&spage=S27&pages=S27-S28&date=2015&title=Internation
al+Psychogeriatrics&atitle=Promoting+social+health+for+people+affected+by+dementi
a%3A+An+online+module+for+National+Health+Service+staff&aulast=Downs
https://ucl-new-primo.hosted.exlibrisgroup.com/openurl/UCL/UCL_VU2?sid=OVID:psyc
db&id=pmid:&id=doi:10.1111%2Fj.1532-5415.2004.52058.x&issn=0002-8614&isbn=
&volume=52&issue=2&spage=195&pages=195-204&date=2004&title=Journal+of+the
+American+Geriatrics+Society&atitle=Incidence+and+Prevalence+of+Dementia+in+th
e+Cardiovascular+Health+Study.&aulast=Fitzpatrick
Jenkins, R. (1997). *Rethinking Ethnicity: Arguments and Explorations*. London: SAGE.
Jenkins, R. (2008). *Rethinking Ethnicity*. London: SAGE.
Jenkins, R. (2014). *Social Identity*. Abingdon: Routledge.
Jivraj, S. (2012). How has ethnic diversity grown 1991-2001-2011. *Manchester: Centre on Dynamics of Ethnicity (CoDE)*, University of Manchester.
Katz, M. J., Lipton, R. B., Hall, C. B., Zimmerman, M. E., Sanders, A. E., Verghese, J., Dickson, D. W., & Derby, C. A. (2012). Age-specific and sex-specific prevalence and incidence of mild cognitive impairment, dementia, and Alzheimer dementia in blacks and whites: A report from the Einstein Aging Study. *Alzheimer Disease & Associated Disorders*, *26*(4), 335–343.
Kirk, D. H., & Goon, S. (1975). Desegregation and the cultural deficit model: An examination of the literature. *Review of Educational Research*, *45*(4), 599–611.
Knapp, M., Prince, M., Albanese, E., Banerjee, S., Dhanasiri, S., & Fernandez, J. (2007). Dementia UK: The full report. London: Alzheimer's Society.
Leibing, A. (2018). Situated prevention: Framing the 'new dementia'. *Journal of Law, Medicine & Ethics*, *46*(3), 704–716.
Lin, S. S., & Kelsey, J. L. (2000). Use of race and ethnicity in epidemiologic research: concepts, methodological issues, and suggestions for research. *Epidemiologic Reviews*, *22*(2), 187–202.
Lipsedge, M., & Littlewood, R. (2005). *Aliens and Alienists: Ethnic Minorities and Psychiatry*. London: Routledge.
Malik, K. (1996). *The Meaning of Race: Race, History and Culture in Western Society*. New York: Macmillan International Higher Education.
Manly, J. J. (2005). Advantages and disadvantages of separate norms for African Americans. *The Clinical Neuropsychologist*, *19*(2), 270–275.
Manly, J. J. (2006). Deconstructing race and ethnicity: Implications for measurement of health outcomes. *Medical Care*, *44*, S10–S16.
McKenney, N. R., & Bennett, C. E. (1994). Issues regarding data on race and ethnicity: The Census Bureau experience. *Public Health Reports*, *109*(1), 16.
Mehta, K. M., & Yeo, G. W. (2017). Systematic review of dementia prevalence and incidence in United States race/ethnic populations. *Alzheimer's & Dementia*, *13*(1), 72–83.
Miles, R. (2004). *Racism*. London: Routledge.
Montagu, A. (1942). Man's most dangerous myth: The fallacy of race. *Man's most dangerous myth: The fallacy of race*.
Moore, J. H. (2008). *Encyclopedia of Race and Racism*. New York: Macmillan Reference USA.
Moriarty, J., Sharif, N., & Robinson, J. (2011). *Black and minority ethnic people with dementia and their access to support and services*. http://www.scie.org.uk/publications/briefings/files/briefing35.pdf
Mukadam, N., Cooper, C., & Livingston, G. (2013). Improving access to dementia services for people from minority ethnic groups. *Current Opinion in Psychiatry*, *26*(4), 409–414. https://doi.org/10.1097/YCO.0b013e32835ee668

Mukadam, N., Waugh, A., Cooper, C., & Livingston, G. (2015). *What would encourage help-seeking for memory problems among UK-based South Asians? A qualitative study.*

Neblett Jr, E. W. (2019). Racism and health: Challenges and future directions in behavioral and psychological research. *Cultural Diversity and Ethnic Minority Psychology, 25*(1), 12.

Predelli, L. N., Halsaa, B., Thun, C., & Sandu, A. (2012). *Majority-Minority Relations in Contemporary Women's Movements: Strategic Sisterhood.* Basingstoke: Palgrave Macmillan.

Prince, M., Knapp, M., Guerchet, M., McCrone, P., Prina, M., Comas-Herrera, A., Wittenberg, R., Adelaja, B., Hu, B., & King, D. (2014). Dementia UK: update. *Alzheimer's Society.*

Rai, T., Hinton, L., McManus, R. J., & Pope, C. (2022). What would it take to meaningfully attend to ethnicity and race in health research? Learning from a trial intervention development study. *Sociology of Health & Illness, 44*, 57–72.

Roche, M., Higgs, P., Aworinde, J., & Cooper, C. (2021). A review of qualitative research of perception and experiences of dementia among adults from Black, African, and Caribbean background: What and whom are we researching? *The Gerontologist, 61*(5), e195–e208.

Saeed, A., Rae, E., Neil, R., Connell-Hall, V., & Munro, F. (2020, 2020-06-25). *To BAME or not to BAME: the problem with racial terminology in the civil service.* @CSWnews. https://www.civilserviceworld.com/news/article/to-bame-or-not-to-bame-the-problem-with-racial-terminology-in-the-civil-service

Salkind, N. J. (2008). *Encyclopedia of Educational Psychology.* Thousand Oaks: SAGE Publications.

Scarman, L. S. B. (1986). *The Scarman report: The Brixton disorders 10–12 April 1981: report of an inquiry.* Puffin.

Seabrooke, V., Seabrook, V., & Milne, A. (2004). *Culture and care in dementia: A study of the Asian community in North West Kent.* Alzheimer's and Dementia Support Services.

Senior, P. A., & Bhopal, R. (1994). Ethnicity as a variable in epidemiological research. *BMJ, 309*(6950), 327–330.

Signoret, J.-L., & Hauw, J.-J. (1991). *Maladie d'Alzheimer et autres démences.* Flammarion médecine-sciences.

Sims-Schouten, W., & Gilbert, P. (2022). Revisiting 'resilience' in light of racism, 'othering' and resistance. *Race & Class, 64*, 84–94.

Smedley, A., Takezawa, Y. I., & Wade, P. (2017). Race: Human. *Encyclopædia Britannica. Encyclopædia Britannica Inc.* Retrieved, 22, https://www.britannica.com/topic/race-human.

Solorzano, D. G. (1992). An exploratory analysis of the effects of race, class, and gender on student and parent mobility aspirations. *The Journal of Negro Education, 61*(1), 30–44.

Soy, A. (2020). *Coronavirus in Africa: Five reasons why Covid-19 has been less deadly than elsewhere.* Retrieved 12 April, from https://www.bbc.co.uk/news/world-africa-54418613

Tishkoff, S. A., & Kidd, K. K. (2004). Implications of biogeography of human populations for 'race' and medicine. *Nature Genetics, 36*(11), S21–S27.

Torres, S. (2019). *Ethnicity and Old Age: Expanding Our Imagination.* Bristol: Policy Press.

Torres, S. (2020). Racialization without racism in scholarship on old age. *Swiss Journal of Sociology, 46*(2), 331–349.

UKDRI. (2022). *Diversity and dementia: How is research reducing health disparities?* (Diversity and Dementia, Issue. https://ukdri.ac.uk/uploads/UK-DRI_Dementia_Health_Inequalities_Report_2022.pdf

Washington, H. A. (2006). *Medical Apartheid: The Dark History of Medical Experimentation on Black Americans from Colonial Times to the Present.* New York: Doubleday Books.

Werner, P., Mittelman, M. S., Goldstein, D., & Heinik, J. (2012). Family stigma and caregiver burden in Alzheimer's disease. *Gerontologist, 52*(1), 89–97. Doi: 10.1093/geront/gnr117

Williams, D. R. (1997). Race and health: basic questions, emerging directions. *Annals of Epidemiology, 7*(5), 322–333.

Williams, D. R., Lavizzo-Mourey, R., & Warren, R. C. (1994). The concept of race and health status in America. *Public Health Reports, 109*(1), 26.

Witchalls, C. (2021). *The impact of COVID-19 has been lower in Africa. We explore the reasons.* Retrieved 12 April, from https://theconversation.com/the-impact-of-covid-19-has-been-lower-in-africa-we-explore-the-reasons-164955

Wohland, P., Rees, P., Norman, P., Boden, P., & Jasinska, M. (2010). *Ethnic population projections for the UK and local areas, 2001–2051.* University of Leeds. Retrieved 10 April 2011, from http://www.geog.leeds.ac.uk/fileadmin/downloads/school/research/projects/migrants/WP_ETH_POP_PROJECTIONS.pdf

Part IV
Methodologies

9 'Whose story is it and what is it for?'

Life story as critical discourse in dementia studies

Jackie Kindell, Aagje Swinnen, and John Keady

Introduction

As a part of biographical approaches to ageing, life story work is deeply embedded in dementia studies and is performed in domestic and care settings. Life story work has been described as being instrumental to 'doing' person-centred care and it is intertwined with many engagement approaches familiar to practitioners in the field, such as reminiscence and formulation activities. In many ways, undertaking life story work compensates for the everyday challenges a person living with dementia often faces and acts as a guardian in preserving a person's sense of identity and selfhood (this responds to the psychosocial scholarships described by Fletcher in Chapter 1). Nowadays, the performance and recording of a life story is often seen as a measure of 'good practice' by professional bodies regulating care practices for people living with dementia and many paper, electronic (apps) and digital documents exist to help in that recording process. Whilst these are all important developments, this chapter takes a step back and focusses instead on the debates and dilemmas that sit behind the act of 'doing' life story work with/alongside people living with dementia. By following this approach, we hope to tease out some of the ethical, practical, practice, moral and emotional investment necessary to undertake life story work. Moreover, whilst the space in the chapter does not allow us to answer the questions we ourselves raise through the direction of our conversation, we hope that some of the captured points are seen as the start of a critical discourse on the subject matter, rather than as an end-point in themselves.

By means of context, the authors of this chapter have worked in, and around, dementia care for a number of years. For example, Jackie, as a highly specialist speech and language therapist in dementia, underpinned her PhD studies by modifying life story work for people with semantic dementia into accessible storylines and developed a new typology where life story work was seen to develop five points of connection: interactional, emotional, new, practical and future (Kindell et al., 2019); Aagje has examined representations of dementia experiences in literature and film as well as creative approaches to dementia care based on the spoken word, such as TimeSlips and the Alzheimer's Poetry Project (Swinnen, 2016; Swinnen and de Medeiros, 2018); and John as a mental health nurse has used life story as a method in developing participatory and co-constructed research alongside people

DOI: 10.4324/9781003290353-14

living with dementia (Keady et al., 2007; Williams and Keady, 2021). Jackie and John are based in Manchester in the United Kingdom, whilst Aagie is based in Maastricht in the Netherlands.

Given our physical location in different European countries, in order to develop and produce this chapter we first met on Microsoft Teams at the end of January 2022 for a recorded, unstructured conversation that was organised, and guided, by both editors of this book. That conversation was transcribed through the in-built software as part of Microsoft Teams and the proofed transcription was sub-sequently sent to us by e-mail by the book editors a week or so after our first meeting. As the three-chapter authors, we then met virtually on our own in early February 2022 to reflect upon the contents of the transcript and to begin to explore the conversational content and the inherent meanings and flow that it contained. As the themes began to take shape through our meeting and subsequent email ex-changes (and attachments), we then met virtually on two other occasions to make sure that the emergent themes and their content was an authentic and meaningful representation of our initial conversation and follow-on exchanges. The emergent themes were identified as: (1) entangled life stories; (2) the value and ethics of life story work and (3) future life story work. Our most recent, and final, virtual meeting took place in mid-June 2022 to reach a conclusion to the chapter, which we will present at the end of this text as a series of bullet points. During this final meeting, it also became apparent that, retrospectively, the guiding question of our conversation turned out to be 'Whose story is it and what is it for?' and given its importance, it is this overarching question that we have placed as the prefix to the title of this chapter.

Underpinned by the three descriptive themes and informed by the overarching research question, this chapter is presented as an open conversation between the three of us. We found that this format enabled a more natural and relaxed discourse on life story work to emerge and be communicated. It is to the sharing of these three themes that we will now turn.

Theme 1: Entangled life stories

Setting the scene

Stories are told and shared in an interactional context and become a vehicle to perform identity work and build relationships (the generative power of storytell-ing is unpacked by Hartung in Chapter 5). Storytelling in conversation is not the performance of a monologue but an interactional endeavour: it is, in other words, co-produced. As with all conversation, a variety of activities beyond reporting facts can be achieved, including joking, arguing, telling troubles, complaining, enter-taining, gossiping, conveying pride and so on (Sidnell, 2010). Moreover, the col-laborative nature of social interaction means that participants directly influence each other with the 'in the moment' choices they make. When a person living with dementia has difficulty with communication, the conversation partner can therefore make adjustments to support, or scaffold, the interaction so the person living with dementia can take a more active role (Kindell et al., 2019). Bringing an interactional lens to life story work allows for an exploration of relationships and identity and how these constructs can be created, maintained and performed, not only by the person living with dementia but also by those around them within an 'in the moment' interaction (Keady et al., 2022). This also helps to explain some of the complexities of life story work in dementia care, including how to support those who may have considerable communication difficulties and the emotional dimensions for the person and their family both 'in the moment' and reaching back into the past. In this respect, life story is also a story about time and how time is lived, expressed and experienced. And time is never static (an observation that Capstick emphasises in Chapter 2).

Aagje: I think one of the things that has emerged in life story work from literary scholarship is this idea that a story is always embedded in the master narratives of our society. What comes across as an individual story is always embedded in these larger stories that people relate to. Therefore, when you do life story work, it is important to make yourself sensitive to all the things that are not being said. The silences, basically. We have to become sensitive to the impact of these larger narratives on people's lives and their story work, these values and ideologies that you have to relate to. During processes of transcription and notetaking, narratives become disembodied and distanced from the moment in which they emerged.

Jackie: Removing that interactional context can also sanitise, or even eliminate, the emotional dimensions for those involved and we then have to be careful about making assumptions. Some of the life story work that we may think is about provoking happy memories, like talking about childhood, might for some lead them to relive past trauma. It is also important to consider the perspective of family members, some of whom may find it deeply upsetting to see the person living with dementia unable to communicate about shared recollections that are important to their relationship or appear to have no memory of important events. When we think about life story work as an intervention, we need to be mindful of these things. There is a misconception that you cannot do any damage and the process is always positive, but it is not that simple. A colleague of mine described how, at a musical evening for people living with dementia, a couple got up to dance 'their song' which had been carefully chosen as part of the musical line up for the evening. Staff were impressed the woman living with dementia danced with good rhythm and enjoyed herself, but the husband came off the dance floor in tears as his wife had been unable to do the steps to their dance anymore and, for him, it reinforced his loss.

John: There is the issue of shared knowledge too. If it is your husband or wife or partner, and you have lived with them for a long time, then why would you do a life story? It is likely to be information you already know, so you have to question the rationale for life story work, consider what you hope to achieve by it and explain this to all concerned. There is also an element of ownership of knowledge, ownership of information and the sharing of that information. We also need to consider what the person living with dementia is able to keep to themselves about their life experiences and how they want to represent their own life story. It is finding ways to support the person living with dementia to have more agency and control within the process. We will all have to think creatively about how this could be achieved so that it is not just 'lip service' to this ambition. Perhaps we also need to be thinking about documenting our own life stories throughout our lives so that should we lose capacity at a future time, our life record will be our own creation and public document ... and not simply a set of recycled stories told by others about us.

Jackie: Life story work is not just one thing, it can include lots of different activities and can be done in different ways and recorded in different formats. Sometimes people want something simple and that might be important in certain care settings to make sure people's basic needs are attended to, like the things they like to eat or not, how they like to spend their time and so on. But it is not possible to convey the complexity and richness of the person, their life and their relationships in a very basic format.

Aagje: It reminds me very much of the more critical trend within dementia studies to think of human beings as interdependent in ways that build on, but also depart from, how Tom Kitwood and the scholars that were influenced by his work understood personhood. We have to think of the story, not as a story of an individual, but more as the story of entanglements with other human beings, and from a post-humanist perspective, also with things and our natural surroundings, including animals. Within the context of life story, this can be a way of opening up ideas about whether a person is what they were in the past. We can become much more conscious of what a person can become in new entanglements, in new environments.

Jackie: Part of our research exploring different points of connection in life story work emphasised the potential of the approach to build new connections in new environments and find creative ways to do this. For example, one of the people that we worked with was extremely disabled in terms of his communication, but he had islands of ability as well, like all people living with dementia. One of the things he could do was an upper-class English accent, as well as extravagant gestures and facial expression, which was quite different to his usual accent and manner. Whilst both he and his wife came from a relatively 'ordinary' background, comments from his mother when they married had led to a long-standing family joke that he came from a 'well-to-do family' and he had married beneath that. This recurring family narrative was humorously woven into lots of conversations over the years. When he went to live in a care home, we explained this to the staff and asked them to encourage this skill by starting interactions with him themselves, using this upper-class tone and body language. He would walk around the home and as he encountered staff they would use this to make a social connection with him and he would respond demonstrating this ability which he enjoyed enormously. It is unlikely that this would have been uncovered in a simple questionnaire about the man's life; it needed time to get to know him and his family. And if the staff had not known that about him, then all that interaction, and all that fun, could have been missed. The staff were also amazed he retained this ability and that helped too in how they perceived him. It was a very embodied skill, quite performative. That is where the crossover with performance studies occurs: a repeat performance 'in the moment' linked to the past and with the power to build new relationships with others.

John: For many years when we have done our research alongside people living with an earlier diagnosis of dementia, we have asked the person to share their life story based on Jay Gubrium's work. So, if your life story was a book, what would its chapters be? Where would you start? What would the title of your book be? It is a really lovely way of getting very quickly to a life story created by the person living with dementia. Interestingly, most people living with dementia doing this 'exercise' have listed the chapters of their book chronologically and start in childhood. Very rarely will somebody say: 'Chapter 9, my dementia'. They very seldom talk about that. When we have done a similar technique with people who have had a stroke, most people's Chapter 1 is their stroke because of the huge impact on their life. But in terms of dementia, it is more loosely integrated into life from the person's perspective. Again, this takes time to uncover. It is another part of dementia care or practice which is not something you can do in half an hour and walk away from. It is something that is about commitment and time investment.

Theme 2: The value and ethics of life story work

Setting the scene

What is the value of life story work and how should we determine it? This is one of the topics that we address in this section, (see also Dowlen and Fleetwood-Smith in Chapter 10). Pay attention to our choice of the words *value* and *determine*. We notice an increasing tendency to position life story work as health care *interventions* which *effect* or *impact* need to be *measured* according to standards in medical and health sciences to get recognition and funding (Gridley et al., 2020). We look at this approach as a *transdisciplinary mismatch* given that storytelling is invaluable as an essential characteristic of how human beings interconnect and give meaning to their lives. As such, it is not meant to reduce symptoms or behaviours of people who live with dementia that are perceived as problematic, although it could be a side-effect of course. Instead, an interest in the story behind the person who lives with dementia should be a given which requires a perspective change in some caregivers.

Life story work must not only focus on biographical fact but also on experience 'in the moment' and how it is expressed creatively through imaginative play (Bellass et al., 2019). Awareness that there is no such thing as the *right* story is crucial to make life story work valued, as further addressed under theme 3. This presumes an open-mind and willingness to attune to the different non-verbal communicative capabilities of the person concerned. There are other advantages to life story work as well in that both the underlying process and the creative mediation of its output can help correct inaccurate representations of people living with dementia – representations that not only circulate in the media but also influence the ways in which we approach them. (See discussions by Mason and colleagues in Chapter 3 and the Scottish Dementia Alumni in Chapter 12 regarding how such representations can have negative impacts on the lives of people affected by dementia.)

Jackie: Is life story work an intervention? Sometimes that perspective can be damaging, particularly if the focus becomes about the accuracy of memories rather than the quality of the interaction itself. If you have a family member who states that a story did not happen, or the information is incorrect, the encounter can be upsetting for all concerned. Does it really matter? Well, it might in some circumstances, so you cannot simply say that you always have to go with the flow. But equally, you might feel that there is some room for discussion. Why are they mixing memories? Can you work with what they are saying 'in the moment'? Can you build on that?

Aagje: The focus is so often on *repair*. Especially in early reminiscence work where you have the photo books and then you practice and practice again until you remember your children's names so to speak. This sets the wrong tone and has a huge impact. Still today in caregiving settings this is often what people think they need to do to help the person who lives with dementia, not realising that it is potentially harmful. There are other ways, but for some reason I think this model has become rather predominant.

Jackie: Indeed, it does not have to be about the correct interpretation. Some relatives worry that if the person says the 'wrong' memories, then that it will interfere with them remembering the 'right' memories at another time. Relatives therefore may see a life story resource as aiming to help the person living with dementia to retain memories in order to keep particular memories alive. You can get into this cycle sometimes, whereas actually it can be about supporting the person living with dementia to express themselves and make connections with others. It is not the *transactional* point of the communication, getting the 'facts correct', that really matters. Rather, it is the *interactional* and social point of the communication. It is great to go wherever the conversation takes us, instead of dictating that you have got to remember a certain fact; for example, that we got married in this particular church, in the particular month and so on.

John: Part of the larger narrative is that we are trying to construct ourselves in the act of storytelling. To get those stories you must have the interest to actually document those stories. It is upsetting when people living with dementia are admitted into care environments and all you have is three or four lines about their life and their life experiences.

Jackie: One of the clinicians I work with often produces one-page summaries, but the point that she makes is that these are not done in 10 minutes. These are hours and hours of work to collect important things about this person that are unique to them or that will be important to their care.

John: I first got into dementia care in the April of 1983. I was a first-year mental health nurse student at that time, placed on a psychogeriatric unit in an asylum with 40 men living with dementia. And there was one man there who had moved down from Newcastle-upon-Tyne to be in the East End of London but had never lost his Northeast accent. I may have lost my Geordie accent now, but that is where I am from. In this man's nursing Kardex notes, it said that he talked 'nonsense' all day and could not be understood. Full stop. I sat down next to him and listened. He was talking in a dialect I was familiar with; I could interpret what he was saying and tease out memories through a shared regional identity and knowledge of place. That is very simple life story work, but it had a profound impact on me because he should not have been labelled and written off in the way that he had been. I was 22 in 1983 and I did not understand the broader meanings of what I was seeing or hearing or witnessing, or had been taught anything meaningful to help in my communication skills. Thinking back now, I was exploring and experiencing a sense of disconnection and the inherent value of conducting life story work. That person living with dementia's identity was being undermined on a daily basis, simply because there was no cultural connection to him in the environment in which he was living out his life.

Jackie: I have had situations where people have told me things that no one in their family knows. The burden of that information sometimes is huge. You must think very deeply about what information you put where and how it will be used. Some of the information might be important to help us understand somebody. For example, a person living with dementia who has been abused at some point in their earlier life may be very fearful during intimate personal care tasks, such as washing and dressing. Their past life experience will influence their perception of the situation and their behaviour, particularly as their memory difficulties may mean care staff are experienced as strangers to them. You cannot ignore this information, it is directly relevant to care and how best to help the person. It might have to be noted somewhere – you just have to be careful about where.

We talk about confidentiality in healthcare, and then we come to do life story work and we put everything in a book that then lives on the coffee table in a care home! I have seen staff ask people living with dementia very personal things in open wards, with everybody listening. When you have dementia, your life becomes very public. Some of the ethical debates should consider those elements of control and who has access to slices of your story. A person's life story is not always considered as confidential, and the care and attention to this dimension is not as prominent as it would be in other situations. We would not have a counselling session on a ward with everybody listening. We would not have our psychological therapy in that environment.

Aagje: There is a thin line between therapy and creativity that is based on storytelling and the yard stick of the former is increasingly used to measure the effect of the latter. As a humanities scholar, this is incomprehensible to me. The idea that storytelling and the arts *work* is an assumption underlying everything we do, rather than the other way around. For this reason, I dislike the intervention focus and the emphasis on *positive* health outcomes. The widespread assumption is that it all has to be joy and smiles and laughter. From my observations, value is really in the whole palette of emotions, including trauma, sadness and disappointment that need to be expressed. I think there has to be space for the whole spectrum of emotions as it is part of human life itself.

Theme 3: Future life story work

Setting the scene

Capturing a life story is not a static, once-only event. It is an interactional experience that moves through and over time creating multiple life storylines in the process (Fletcher and Capstick emphasise this multiplicity in the concluding chapter). Indeed, our lives are in a perpetual state of motion and we would suggest that for people living with dementia, it is now possible for life story documentation and practice to take account of new opportunities that are present in our digital age. Indeed, from a Western perspective, it is sobering to think that the average 80-year-old person will have seen technology progress from messages sent and received by telegram at the start of their lives, to the everyday use of the smartphone in contemporary society where conversation can be instantaneous and broadcast quality images can be sent on the same hand-held device through a mobile connection to the internet. The speed of change is breath-taking. That said, technology will continue to evolve and at some point in time, the shiny new smartphone of today will look and feel as obsolete as the telegram does to us now. As we search for constants in an ever-changing world, relationships and opportunities to maintain meaningful relationships are seen by people living with dementia as a foundational aspect of their everyday life (Reilly et al., 2020). In this section, we will reflect on the past to explore the form and content of future life story work and what responsibilities we all have for ensuring relationships matter so that our individual narratives are preserved and shared in an empowered way.

John: Our focus on life story again takes me back to the early 1980s when I first worked as a student mental health nurse on the 'psychogeriatric' wards in the asylum in Essex where I trained. At the time, we would be encouraged to do classroom reality orientation where we would sit people living with dementia in rows of chairs facing a blackboard. The words on the blackboard would just say: *'Today is…'*; *'The weather is…'*; *'The season is…'* and each day we would fill in the blanks with our pieces of chalk and ask people living with dementia to repeat the answers back to us. It was like being back at school. It was well meant, but it did not really serve a meaningful purpose. I think it may be that, in life story work, we are at a similar critical juncture where what was once accepted as good practice, in reality needs to stop so that we can begin to move forward in a new and different direction.

Aagje: I wonder what kind of convergences we can find between life story work and literary scholarship. A lot has been written about the fact that a life story is not necessarily just an unmediated reflection of an experience. It is a mediated version that is told 'in the moment' and can be retold in many different ways. This has a lot to do with the genre of life story itself. When you ask a person to tell their story as a book with chapters, then from the moment you are born, you learn all these terms of emplotment in the story. You pick all these iconic life moments, such as when you graduate, when you get married, when you have a child, and so on. That type of emplotment can be very normative. It is also very heteronormative in that it assumes that all families include a husband and a wife with children even though this model no longer reflects the reality of the different types of families and kinship people develop, such as when we think of newly composed families, trans families, one-person households, and so on. We have to be more creative in how we ask people to make these stories. For instance, if you ask people to think of a moment of great difficulty and how they handled it, then a very different type of life story is told.

Jackie: The assumptions that we make in daily life carry into dementia care. All of those things, all of those cultural prejudices, are there too. There are lots of different life story templates available, but they all tend to follow the same format: 'Where were you born?'; 'Where did you get married?'; 'Where did you work?' and so on. Some of these events the person may never have experienced. I like to start with a blank piece of paper and encourage the person to talk about what is important to them or find other ways to stimulate connections. I find it much more free-flowing than simply 'filling in my life story sheet'.

John: I am coming to the end of my career probably knowing much less about dementia now than I did when I started. I think you go through an evolving process, realising that people living with dementia are much more than clinical objects. As Tom Kitwood said in his *Dementia Reconsidered* book, if you want to do person centred care, then you must start with life story work because it is foundational to the approach. In developing a new critical discourse on life story work in dementia, there is also something about the accompanying development of creative methods as well. In our research work over the years alongside people living with dementia, we have used video, photography, object identification, animation, cameras, drawings and so on. Anything that can support the empowerment and communication of that person living with dementia is important to us. But is that just everyday practice in a different guise?

Aagje: Critical dementia studies should not forget what happened in the 1990s. We just have to take the initial work on personhood further. The work of Tom Kitwood and Steven Sabat was really eye-opening at the time; the whole idea of the *person* behind the illness of dementia, of personhood as something that needs to be upheld by others. But since then, different conceptualisations of 'the person' and subject formation have been called on to better understand what dementia signifies. We have realised that a person is not only relational but also embodied and performative and that identity is constantly in flux. I think that for the sake of politics and ethics we have to take dementia scholarship a step further, to move ever further away of the neuropsychiatric biopolitics of dementia. In the ethnographic work that I have been doing, what I feel are the most important moments are when the 'norm' of able-bodiedness and able-mindedness is questioned to such an extent that you, yourself, understand that maybe you are not the 'norm'. These are the most empowering moments, when self-identity is questioned. It is not when we keep trying to see the person behind the illness or when we try to establish a kind of 'permanent personhood'. We need some type of activism that is not only about inclusion and participation but is a much more radical rethinking of the world and our society and how we want to live with, and as, older people.

John: In semantic dementia, where Jackie continues to work, there was no research in life story work prior to her starting her PhD study. Part of our own frustration and way of thinking at the time was that we needed to push new boundaries and try to reconstruct new narratives and new stories about the 'here and now' that embrace the future for people with semantic dementia. One that was built from remembered life storylines.

Aagje: This ties in with play and improvisation, not in a professional way, but in an everyday way. If life is a stage, then this is exactly what we do all day long, we just have to learn to tap into it in our interaction. Whilst truth telling may be important in certain circumstances, in others less so, or even not at all. I lean more towards the idea of imagination. I can understand that for family members it may be devastating to suddenly hear that your partner was married to someone else or living in a different place – even if this never happened of course. But for the 'here and now' and for the future, does it really matter?

Personally, I feel that there has to be room for something else and something new. It comes back to a hermeneutical stance, to search for something and to take it seriously rather than to correct it. To me, everything that the person says should be taken seriously in order to put the pieces together and try to figure out what is really going on. There is a deeper truth to things that you have to discover. That is actually also how I want people to treat me.

Conclusion

This chapter is meant to ask questions of the readership. We do not pretend, or even claim, to hold the answers to some of the issues that we have raised in our conversation; they are simply *our experiences* and *our reflections* of being involved in life story work alongside people living with dementia, families and practitioners over a number of years. That said, in the Introduction to this chapter, we shared that our most recent, and final, virtual meeting took place in mid-June 2022 to reach a conclusion to our chapter by reflecting on our time together on the project. At that meeting we decided to present our exchanged thoughts as a series of bullet points, which we will now share as follows:

- Eliciting a life story in a dementia care setting serves as: (i) a means for the person who lives with dementia to express themselves and give meaning to their lives; (ii) an interpretative framework for present behaviour that is perceived as difficult to understand and (iii) as a tool to sustain relations (with family members and friends) and even create new ones (with caregivers, new material environments).
- The personhood movement in dementia research and practice has put great emphasis on the importance of the life story to uphold the identity of the person living with dementia and the responsibility of their surroundings to 'bestow it upon' them, as Kitwood (1997) himself phrased it. This idea is still the basis of much dementia scholarship even though it is now contested because of the implied power imbalance (discussed by Fletcher in Chapter 1).
- The phrasing 'bestowing personhood' and the view behind it, unintentionally risks continuing an 'us' (able-minded people) and 'them' (neurodivergent people) dialectic that may result in social injustices against people who live with dementia (positioned as lost selves in need of saving interventions). In life story work, this comes to the fore when life story facilitators insist on 'getting the facts right' and/or do not honour the sensitivity and privacy of the story shared.
- Recent post-humanist perspectives in critical dementia studies (outlined by Lotherington in Chapter 6 and Williamson and Jenkins in Chapter 11), help us move beyond this binary by addressing how all humans are fundamentally

entangled with other humans and non-humans and how this entanglement is constantly up for change and negotiation – what Haraway (2008) calls a lateral 'becoming with'.

- Translated to life story work in dementia care, this implies that just like human beings change in interaction with their environment, stories are constantly in flux. Of course, we do acknowledge that people who live with dementia change in ways that are not only unexpected, but often also experienced as problematic. Honouring change is not meant to ignore the often-complex reality of long-term care, but can introduce some important temporal perspective on change, (see Capstick in Chapter 2).
- Theory and practice often develop at a different pace. Much of our conversation is still focused on how we can make people (not just those involved in dementia care but in society at large) understand that there still is a person behind the dementia diagnosis. Acknowledging personhood is then a first step towards the realisation of compassionate dementia care (Treadaway et al., 2019). Only when the person is acknowledged, can we start discussing how they and their stories change – just like anybody else's – and be open to the surprise and wonder new encounters can bring.
- Life story work is also about the future as well as the past. As such, the focus on reminiscence activities and life review as 'go to' contexts for life story work may well needs to be fundamentally re-thought and re-appraised.

References

Bellass, S., Balmer, A., May, V., Keady, J., Buse, C., Capstick, A.J., Burke, L., Bartlett, R. and Hodgson, J. (2019). Broadening the debate on creativity and dementia: A critical approach. *Dementia: The International Journal of Social Research and Practice*, 18(7–8): 2799–2820.

Gridley, K., Birks, Y. F. and Parker, G. M. (2020). Exploring good practice in life story work with people with dementia: The findings of a qualitative study looking at the multiple views of stakeholders. *Dementia: The International Journal of Social Research and Practice*, 19(2): 182–194.

Haraway, D. (2008). *When species meet*. Minnesota: University of Minnesota Press.

Keady, J., Campbell, S., Clark, A., Dowlen, R., Elvish, R., Jones, L., Kindell, J., Swarbrick, S. and Williams, S. (2022). Re-thinking and re-positioning 'being in the moment' within a continuum of moments: introducing a new conceptual framework for dementia studies. *Ageing & Society*, 42: 681–702.

Keady, J., Williams, S. and Hughes-Roberts, J. (2007). 'Making Mistakes': using Co-Constructed Inquiry to illuminate meaning and relationships in the early adjustment to Alzheimer's disease – a single case study approach. *Dementia: The International Journal of Social Research and Practice*, 6(3): 343–364.

Kindell, J., Wilkinson, R. and Keady, J. (2019). From conversation to connection: a cross-case analysis of life story work with five couples where one partner has semantic dementia. *Ageing & Society*, 39(10): 2322–2345.

Kitwood, T. (1997). *Dementia reconsidered: The person comes first*. Maidenhead: Open University Press.

Reilly, S.T., Harding, A.J.E., Morbey, H., Ahmed, F., Williamson, P.R., Swarbrick, C., Leroi, I., Davies, L., Reeves, D., Holland, F., Hann, M. and Keady, J. (2020). What is important to people with dementia living at home? A set of core outcome items for use in the evaluation of non-pharmacological community-based health and social care interventions. *Age and Ageing*, 49(4): 664–671.

Sidnell, J. (2010). *Conversation analysis: An introduction.* Chichester, West Sussex: Wiley-Blackwell.

Swinnen, A. (2016). Healing words: Critical inquiry of poetry interventions in dementia care. *Dementia: The International Journal of Social Research and Practice*, 15(6): 1377–1404.

Swinnen, A. and de Medeiros, K. (2018). "Play" and people living with dementia: A humanities-based inquiry of TimeSlips and the Alzheimer's Poetry Project. *The Gerontologist*, 58(2): 261–269.

Treadaway, C., Taylor, A. and Fennell, J. (2019). Compassionate design for dementia care. *International Journal of Design Creativity and Innovation*, 7(3): 144–157.

Williams, S. and Keady, J. (Eds.) (2021). *Participatory case study work: Approaches, authenticity and application in ageing studies.* London: Routledge.

10 From symptoms to citizenship

A critical reading of the perceived value of arts and culture in a dementia context

Robyn Dowlen and Rebecka Fleetwood-Smith

Introduction

There has been a growing narrative of the positive value of the creative arts in the context of dementia over the past twenty years. There is a wide range of literature that showcases the broad nature of arts and cultural engagement in the context of dementia, including (but not limited to): visits to museums and galleries (Camic et al., 2019); 'dementia friendly' cinema screenings (Broome et al., 2020); music programmes led by professional orchestral musicians (Dowlen et al., 2022); devising theatrical performances centred on storytelling (Basting et al., 2016); as well as online music-making via Zoom during the Covid-19 crisis (Dowson et al., 2021). Alongside research in this area which has reported on the positive value of arts and cultural engagement for people living with dementia (e.g. Zeilig et al., 2014; Dowson et al., 2021; Kinsey et al., 2021), there has also been growing advocacy for access to such experiences (e.g. All-Party Parliamentary Group on Arts, Health and Wellbeing, 2017; Bowell & Bamford, 2018; Tapson et al., 2018; UK Music & Music for Dementia, 2021).

While this area of research and practice has seen significant growth in recent years, we have observed a lack of criticality applied to understanding the value of the arts in the context of dementia. Although there has been growing critique surrounding the ways in which the impacts of arts-based programmes can be 'measured' – i.e. before and after approaches within time-limited 'interventions' (see Dowlen et al., 2022) – there has been little attention paid to the narratives that underpin the use of the arts in this context, or the ways in which the arts could contribute to the stigmatisation of people living with dementia. In this chapter, we unpack some of these critiques and consider what they mean for this area of research and practice going forward.

To begin, we want to make it apparent that we approach this topic area as two cisgender, white, non-disabled women, from middle-class backgrounds, who have had the opportunities to engage with arts and culture across our childhoods and our adulthood. We both come from backgrounds in psychology and the arts – Robyn being a trained musician in two instruments and chartered psychologist; and Rebecka with a background in textile design and applied psychology. We recognise that through the privileges afforded by our backgrounds we have not experienced

DOI: 10.4324/9781003290353-15

the systemic barriers that limit access to arts and cultural experiences to many people. Furthermore, we work with a range of creative practitioners and cultural organisations who advocate for the 'power' of arts and culture in the lives of people with dementia. However, we recognise that there is a lack of criticality that has been applied to this field to date (Zeilig et al., 2014) – with the assumption that the arts are inherently beneficial to all people with dementia, without consideration of the theoretical, societal and political structures surrounding the opportunities for such experiences. In this chapter, we therefore present our reading of arts and dementia literature alongside illustrations drawn from our own reflective accounts of working in this field over the past eight years. This chapter will not seek to provide a synthesis of research findings in this area as this has been done extensively elsewhere (see for example: Van der Steen et al., 2018; Letrondo et al., 2022) but rather we explore this work more broadly within a critical framing.

Narratives of decline: Over-Medicalising creative experiences?

In order to critically explore the arts within the context of dementia we must consider the (bio)medical model of dementia which sees the condition described as a 'disease' and perceived as a loss of 'normality' (ideas critiqued by Fletcher in Chapter 1). In practice, this has led to dementia being seen as something to be diagnosed and treated, involving, for instance, the management of 'difficult' behaviours, resulting in people living with the condition becoming 'victims' and 'sufferers' (see Mason and colleagues' discussion of these terms in Chapter 3). The detrimental effects of this language alone are evident in the accounts of members of the Dementia Engagement and Empowerment Project in Chapter 3. The impact that the medicalisation of the condition has on those living with dementia should not be underestimated as Shakespeare et al. (2019) write:

> A person with dementia ends up being treated as dependent and denied a voice. Perhaps a better extrapolation of what happens when someone has dementia is that she is viewed in terms of her inabilities, whether these are cognitive, relational or functional, and in comparison to an expected norm of personhood. Her strength becomes invisible. Her emotional and social bonds stand for nothing. Her disease and difficulties become her defining features.
>
> (p. 1082)

This medicalisation of dementia has shaped the ways in which arts and cultural experiences are framed, positioned and often experienced by those with the condition. We see many narratives in this area that over-medicalise and 'interventionalise' creative practices, reducing the experiences of people living with dementia down to the 'problematic' symptoms they exhibit (Kindell and colleagues caution against this interventionalisation in Chapter 9). For example, it is commonplace for cultural experiences to be framed using medical language – something we see both in research and the media. Take for example a 2021 piece published in the guardian 'Alzheimer's patients and hospital staff prescribed music in NHS trial'

(Booth, 2021). In this article, the author uses highly medicalised language to describe the hospital-based programme centred on personalised music playlists, such as:

> The technology operates as a musical "drip", playing songs to patients and monitoring their heart rates as they listen. A 90-year-old might be prescribed big band music, while a 50-year-old might get a dose of Van Halen and Paul McCartney.

The use of the terms 'musical drip', 'dose' and 'prescription' strongly positions this article within the (bio)medical language that is so often used in a dementia context. This narrative ties in with an assumption within (bio)medicalisation of dementia that the arts are something that can be administered like a pharmaceutical drug (de Medeiros & Basting, 2014).

Within research literature to date, creative and cultural experiences have largely been framed as interventions aimed at reducing the so-called 'behavioural and psychological symptoms of dementia' (James & Jackman, 2017). Here, the creative arts are considered as 'interventions' of which success, or failure, which is measured against a reduction of these 'symptoms', such as a lessening of the signs of agitation following a time-limited arts-based intervention (de Medeiros & Basting, 2014). Studies that have used this approach to date have shown mixed findings, with a large number showing no significant reductions in 'symptoms' such as agitation or anxiety (Van der Steen et al., 2018). This has led to the dismissal of many of the positive findings associated with arts-based programmes in the context of dementia, with approaches that do not use standardised outcomes within randomised designs deemed to lack rigour or methodological quality (Gray et al., 2018).

While such pre-post intervention approaches are reasonably typical within (bio) medical approaches to dementia research, it limits the inclusion of the voices of people living with dementia and relies heavily on the second-hand reporting of symptom severity by family members or formal carers. This has led to researchers questioning whether we are missing valuable parts of the lived experiences of people living with dementia by only using pre-post intervention measures given the range of positive benefits that have been observed anecdotally and reported by people living with dementia themselves. For example, Gray et al. (2018) suggest a scarcity in the field of arts and dementia of 'the assessment of artistic quality, aesthetic experience, cultural contributions, process, social impact and economic value' (p. 776). Thus, the (bio)medical model has infiltrated the ways in which the benefits of the arts are perceived in the context of dementia in terms of understanding or 'measuring' its impacts, yet the model permeates further into wider narratives of the arts in the lives of people with dementia.

Overall, the ways in which arts and cultural experiences have been over-medicalised have serious implications for how we seek to understand their impacts in the context of dementia. It has resulted in a lack of focus on people with dementia as artists and creators and reduces their experiences to the 'symptoms' they do or do not exhibit. Next we turn to exploring the universalisation of arts-based practices in the context of dementia, and the challenges surrounding access to arts and cultural experiences.

Assumed homogeneity: Arts for all?

The notion that the arts can be administered like a pharmaceutical drug (de Medeiros & Basting, 2014) not only flattens the arts to an intervention, devoid of its inherent nuance and subjectivity (as discussed in the previous section), but it also implies that people with dementia are a homogeneous group (see Lotherington on strengthening commitments to intersectionality in Chapter 6). The reductionism of people with dementia occurs at many different levels. The portrayals of people with dementia within TV and film reinforce the ways in which people are positioned as a homogeneous group, with people with dementia often depicted as white, female, middle class, living at home (Capstick et al., 2015; also Ludwin in Chapter 7), and we typically 'see' them through the eyes of the caregiver. Capstick et al's (2015) work demonstrates that 'viewing' a person with dementia in this way may mean that their identity is reduced to their diagnosis. This assumed homogeneity often extends into research and practice surrounding the ways in which people with dementia can engage with the arts.

To begin, it is important to acknowledge that not every person with dementia has equal access to the arts and cultural experiences we have discussed earlier in this chapter. We know that there are inequalities more broadly in society when it comes to arts and cultural participation (Mak et al., 2020) and this permeates into the arts and dementia landscape. In the arts and dementia literature we see a homogeneous group represented within research studies (typically older white women with dementia) with questions of barriers to access rarely considered. While well intentioned, arts and cultural 'provision' for people with dementia can miss the mark when it comes to a diverse and inclusive offer in practice too (see Roche and colleagues' critique of the 'cultural' problems targeted by the race and ethnicity scholarship in Chapter 8). For example, in the Baring Foundation's (2019) report: 'Art and dementia in the UK South Asian Diaspora' they explored what kind of arts and cultural activities are meaningful for people living with dementia and detailed the ways in musical activities can alienate people and be a barrier for access, as the quote below highlights:

> People I know and have met, they wouldn't take necessarily well to music or Bollywood type music or dancing, which is why Alzheimer's Society's Memory Cafés don't work well. You have singing and dancing and my mum who has dementia, I wouldn't take her there, she would stick out like a sore thumb. It's not her cultural reference point.
>
> (p. 27)

This draws parallels with Conroy's (2009) critique of creative tensions between drama, theatre and disability arts in which they examine how identifying as disabled is:

> a counter hegemonic act which challenges wider mainstream culture. The organisation of a category of disability, and the formulation of a position of disability oppression moves people from many specific cultures into one

large and universally oppressed category. There is a move from the recognition of cultural differences to a huge belief in a common oppression and denigration of disability.

(p. 3)

Within music practices, there are songs that are almost synonymous with people with dementia and social care settings – Vera Lynne's 'We'll Meet Again', 'Oh Danny Boy'. While there are many shared references that can be drawn upon from these pieces of music, they have the potential to both neglect the cultural backgrounds and ages of those who are engaging, with it being noted that they could be outdated and even patronising (Akhtar et al., 2017). In a recent report published by the (UK government), All-Party Parliamentary Group on Dementia (2022), music is named as an approach to supporting culturally sensitive person-centred care for people with dementia (p. 36). However, as has been discussed, the music and the arts more broadly have the potential to be, at worst exclusionary if they are not culturally grounded and accessible to more than a limited demographic.

Homogeneity within this context also extends to notions that the arts are 'beneficial' for all people with dementia within all contexts. In our experiences, this is truly not the case. This overly positive framing has the potential to be highly problematic in practice as RD illustrates within the following reflection (an experience likely to resonate with those working in arts and dementia):

I remember visiting a care home as I had been invited to observe a music group. In the corner of the room sat a man who had a look of discomfort on his face. He was shouting 'get me out of here'. I watched this man try to get out of the chair he had been placed in, in an environment where he was clearly uncomfortable. I was told by the musicians that this man could not walk by himself and I had no training in physically assisting this person out of the room - so I sought help. I was told by care staff that his expression of wanting to leave the room was just a symptom of his dementia (agitation), and that listening to the music was 'good for him'. In this moment I felt helpless – this man was clearly indicating that he did not want to be in this space but the narrative that music was universally beneficial kept him in the room. He had no agency, he had no choice, the value of music in that moment was decided for him, rather than considering whether it was right for him.

From this example we can see that the perception of the arts, as 'universally good' and an intervention to receive, can in some cases lead to the control and containment of people with dementia. This control shapes the delivery of such 'prescribed' activities, the time, place, setting and context in which they occur (Dowlen & Keady, forthcoming). This application of the arts as some sort of antidote sees the arts often treated with an other-worldly reverence. Whereby we see frequent national and international examples that claim that listening to music 'brought a person back' or that a person 'came alive' when listening to a piece of music (see for example: Moisse, 2012; Dodd, 2018). These perspectives are typically grounded in reminiscence focussed approaches which, although techniques vary, centre on provoking memories (see for example: Macleod et al., 2021; and also Kindell and colleagues in Chapter 9). Such approaches are potentially disorienting and distressing for people with dementia – drawing us to question who these activities are for. Moreover, to view the arts as capable of provoking magical, supernatural moments negates the care, craft and time involved in creativity. For example, De Nora (2017, p. 96) argues that such 'magical' moments are not born from the supernatural, they are made up of ordinary acts which are the product of sensitive, nurturing, relational practices. This notion that the arts are magical draws parallels with disability research which warns against the 'counter-cultural fascination with specific representations/portrayals' of the arts experiences of people with learning disabilities, claiming that a label of 'specialness' is highly problematic and othering and sees people treated as passive receivers of an 'intervention'.

Overall, this section has illustrated how assumptions of homogeneity of the dementia experience impact the ways in which people can access arts and cultural experiences. This has had significant impacts on the way in which the value of arts and cultural experiences has been evaluated and researched in this area. Many reviews that bring together research in this area show limited benefits of different arts and cultural programmes (see for example: Van der Steen et al., 2018; Letrondo et al., 2022) and argue that the heterogeneity of programmes and outcome measures lead to an impossibility when it comes to generalising findings. But should we perhaps be examining arts and cultural experiences from a place of intimate, individual creative experiences rather than attempting to generalise to a group that is assumed to be homogeneous?

Towards creative citizenship?

Throughout history, the arts have been used as a way to explore, process and critique existential questions (European Union Agency for Fundamental Rights, 2017). The provocative capacity of the arts and the ways in which artists are upheld for their ability to tackle and uncover the most challenging and controversial aspects of humanity is not something that is typically acknowledged within the arts and dementia literature. The arts can offer routes with which to explore and express what it is to feel anger, joy, pain, loss, shame, disgust, desire, love and passion. The arts are divisive, subjective and inherently invite critique.

The arts within dementia, despite increasingly being given a certain degree of gravitas (e.g. the magical power of the arts – De Nora, 2017), are not afforded that freedom. The context of dementia and the underlying, pervasive veil of the (bio) medical model curtails, shapes and produces experiences that are at odds with the opportunities that engaging with the arts can afford. If we look at disability studies we see authors critique how disability arts, in line with the individual model of disability, were underpinned by approaches centred on 'normalisation'/'rehabilitation' (Leighton, 2009). In the context of dementia, the arts are positioned as 'curative'/an 'elixir' or a tool in the 'fight against dementia'. This argument corresponds with the ways in which arts and cultural engagement have been (and often continue to be) positioned for people with dementia as a method with which to alleviate symptoms, to occupy individuals and to provide positive (often cited as 'therapeutic') benefits.

Shifting focus away from the arts as an intervention can be powerful for people with dementia. The arts can provide a route for people to express themselves in different ways, as Bartlett (2015) reflects:

> I remember feeling surprised during the first creative workshop when a participant wrote in large red letters on her piece of paper the word, 'underdog'; I had no idea this participant felt so strongly about her perceived lack of status even though I had interviewed her and read her diary.
>
> (p. 761)

A further example demonstrates how creating poetry allowed space for people with dementia to tackle a subject matter that may be perceived as 'risky' for people with dementia (Amponsem et al., 2022). The work, which explored how people with dementia expressed a sense of hope, demonstrated the complex and varied lived experiences of people with the condition. For example, in 'Poem Twenty-Eight' a person expressed the disabling narrative that they are subjected to and conveyed a want to be acknowledged and valued:

> Do we have a goal? Or we have a wish. Do we have a dream? Or we have a faith. No, we have dementia!
>
> End of story here! Yes?

There are also examples where the arts have been used as part of dementia activism, challenging the structures that exclude people with dementia from an active life. For example, a series of banners created by people with dementia as part of The Unfurlings (n.d.) project which drew on the role of banners in highlighting inequalities, and campaigning. The banners (see https://theunfurlings.org.uk/) are statement pieces grounded in the group's campaigning for better support and understanding of dementia by public transport providers. The quotes below are taken from theunfurlings.org.uk:

> 'The banner has two versions a negative side (everything that is wrong with the transport systems and a positive side (how it should be)'.

> 'The colour red symbolises positivity and revolution'.

> 'The embellishments are stylised representations of the roads and railways they are easy to navigate and take a direct route'.

The arts thus appear to provide a platform for citizenship enabling people living with dementia to feel more connected to themselves, to other people, and the sensory world around them. For example, Dupuis et al. (2016) explored citizenship narratives through a participatory arts programme, claiming that engagement with creative practice can be a vehicle with which to exercise citizenship and in turn result in personal and social change. This notion of connectivity was highlighted by Basting (2006), when describing the value of the arts for people living with dementia:

> People with dementia who have edited themselves into silence for fear of saying the wrong thing or shut themselves down to avoid contact they cannot understand, can use the arts to reconnect with themselves and the people who care for them. And perhaps most important, the arts offer a chance for people with dementia to connect with the people who have forgotten them – their communities at large.
>
> (p. 16)

This quote highlights the role of the arts in enabling the inclusion of people living with dementia within their communities and within society more generally. The arts have strong potential to empower people living with dementia to be active citizens, enabling them to shape their own lives and experiences (Dupuis et al., 2016), promoting them to the status of an equal citizen (Bartlett & O'Connor, 2007).

The space created by the arts for intimate self-expression (or indeed activism) is not something that typically defines this area. van der Byl Williams and Zeilig (2022) recently proposed an understanding of agency in dementia as multidimensional, layered and existing on a continuum. Their laminated model presents seven dimensions of agency (i.e. embodied agency, emotional agency, sense of agency, intentional conscious action, social context, decision-making, moral responsibility) and may be instrumental in developing work within arts and dementia. For instance, they use a fictional example of a music making session (drawing on their expertise within working with people with dementia, care workers and creative practitioners) to illustrate how their model could help understand and support the agency of someone with dementia. For example, they describe the ways in which music-making can be an important way for someone to express their emotions and how working within a responsive, participatory framework can 'reaffirm' and help support emotional agency. Their model of agency demonstrates the vast opportunities that the arts can afford people with dementia both in terms of their own personal expression of what it means to live with a diagnosis of dementia, but also opportunities for engaged citizenship and political activism (echoed by the Scottish Dementia Alumni group in Chapter 12).

In a real-world example of this personal expression of what it means to live with dementia, Ronald Amanze (a co-author of Chapter 3) in his talk as part of the Essex Cultural Diversity Project event *Dementia, Diversity and the Arts* (Amanze, 2021) spoke of his experiences of using creative writing to communicate his lifeworld after a diagnosis of dementia following a stroke:

> I actually got to a stage where I literally stopped engaging with the world, and I cut the world off because I wasn't communicating well with the world

and I felt the world just wasn't understanding me. And I started to write about what I felt. Then I started to share it with people. And suddenly they took note of my conversation. People have embraced me more on the conversations I have written in my dementia diaries and more has happened for me from writing my feelings and thoughts using creative expressions then has ever happened for me when I just tried to speak in the norm.

While Amanze (2021) shares his experiences of writing and the ways in which it connects him to the world, we must recognise the complexities involved in carrying out research with people with dementia in this context. For example, researchers are subject to stringent ethical procedures, and while we do not have space to examine these in detail here, such ethical practices place boundaries and contain the very nature of the work (Fletcher, 2021; Campbell et al., in press). In our experiences, ethics boards are far more open to research methodologies more typically associated with (bio)medical approaches to dementia and have questioned whether creative approaches understanding the arts in this context 'count' as research. The rigid structures and frameworks imposed on this work by ethics boards also limit the creative expressions of people with dementia, with contributions having to be anonymised to 'protect' the identities of those involved. Swaffer (2016), who is an academic and campaigner living with young onset dementia, revealed her anger of researchers being cited as the authors of a poem that she wrote, noting that the anonymisation of her (and others') creative contributions neglected 'the creative and intellectual copyright or ownership of people with dementia' (p. 1319). Such constraints arguably limit the extent to which researchers can explore the arts through a lens of relational citizenship as these practices reinforce traditional asymmetric distributions of power.

Within this section, we have examined how the traditional reduction of the arts to an intervention negates the impact that the arts can have in the lives of people with dementia. The arts are not necessarily universally positive but that does not mean that they are not important or of benefit. As we have discussed, the arts can be a way for a person to explore, uncover and express challenging, uncomfortable experiences (Amponsem et al., 2022), for people to engage in activism (Bartlett, 2015) and a way people can exert their agency (van der Byl Williams & Zeilig, 2022). The capacity of the arts is limitless, and this is no less true for the arts in the lives of people with dementia.

Everyday creativity: Magnifying the mundane?

Our discussion so far has largely centred on traditional forms of creative practice (e.g. music, poetry and visual arts) and dementia. Yet, in recent years, researchers have examined notions of everyday creativity within the lives of people with dementia with Bellass et al. (2019) arguing that broadening our understanding of creativity can offer new insights regarding people with the condition and those that surround them. Everyday creativity refers to creativity outside of or beyond traditional forms of creative practice. For example, RFS worked with a person with dementia who said that they would place underwear in public areas of the care home which would cause 'hysteria' (Fleetwood-Smith, 2020):

> The person did not feel that the care home was their home, and this 'disruptive' act was a form of protest. They kept the underwear in their bag on their walking aide and this use of an item immediately close to hand demonstrates a provocative and creative way in which this person expressed themselves.

Attending to everyday creativity necessitates shifting attention from the 'uncovering exceptional' encounters to understanding creativity as central to everyday lives. This shift is more in line with approaches to understanding 'everyday citizenship' in the context of dementia, including the mundane, unremarkable, routine parts of life (Nedlund et al., 2019). Creativity is seen to be a central tenet of the everyday experience of dementia, showcasing how people with dementia are able to exert agency and capacity through their everyday actions. Kontos et al. (2017) centre creativity within their model of 'Relational-Citizenship' which centres on principles of care drawing upon (1) the concept of citizenship, (2) treating the person with dementia as active partners in their care, and (3) embodied selfhood. Kontos' (2004, 2005) work in particular has been instrumental in rethinking selfhood and the role of the body in the context of dementia as it involves considering people with dementia as embodied beings, whose actions, gestures and movements are expressive and relational as opposed to a symptom of the condition. For example, Kontos et al. (2017) refer to an arts programme in which creative practitioners used improvisatory techniques when working with people with dementia as opposed to traditional approaches which centre on 'bringing a person back'.

However, these notions of everyday creativity, and indeed the mundane, do not always sit comfortably with perceptions of how arts and culture can represent a person's dementia experience. For example, in a 2022 episode of *Doing It Right with Pandora Sykes* (Skyes, 2022), Wendy Mitchell (an author and activist living with dementia), stated:

> TV and films they have to sensationalise, they have to get viewers watching. And if they showed the often-mundane reality of living with dementia, it wouldn't grasp the viewer so they have to be dramatic, they believe. They have to be sensationalised. When I was consulted on Casualty – to begin with I was listened to, I felt listened to. The scripts that were coming through represented what I was talking about but as time went on I realised they had stopped listening to me. I actually dropped out of the process, I said I can't be a consultant if you're not going to listen to me.

Mitchell's experience, as shared in the 2022 podcast episode, showcases how public perception of the lived experience of dementia can be skewed through the consumption of popular culture. The 'magical' notion of the arts that we touched upon earlier in this chapter further justifies the need to de-sensationalise people with dementia's experiences with arts, culture and creativity in their everyday lives.

Returning to Kontos et al's (2017) model of relational citizenship, there are new lenses being explored in the context of dementia to examine these everyday instances of creativity which focus on 'in the moment' experiences. Keady and colleagues (2022) define being in the moment as:

> A relational, embodied and multi-sensory human experience. It is both situational and autobiographical and can exist in a fleeting moment or for longer periods of time. All moments are considered to have personal significance, meaning and worth.
>
> (p. 687)

This 'in the moment' lens connects with the ways in which Kontos et al. (2020) explore creative moments and creative practice as deriving from the 'complex intersection of enabling environments and the embodied intentionality of all involved' (p. 1). Thus, as Basting (2020) argues, research around dementia and creativity must move beyond focusing on the individual to exploring relational and everyday aspects of creativity. This necessitates rethinking how dementia is studied and the research methods used (Bellass et al., 2019). As Zeilig et al. (2014) similarly propose, it is maybe not that research is not picking up on the wide and varied benefits of creativity and arts for people with dementia, but that the wrong questions are being asked. A shift towards how people with dementia value the arts, or find meaning in them, may be necessary going forwards to gain more nuanced understandings.

Carrying out research that privileges the everyday lived experiences of people with dementia involves developing a repertoire of approaches (Tsekleves & Keady, 2021). While embracing Bellass et al.'s (2019) broader understanding of creativity arguably involves methods that de-privilege language and involve different ways of engaging with people and environments. For example, researchers working in this area advocate using participatory methods such as photo elicitation, visual and sensory adaptations to interviews and creative research methods (see for example: Buse & Twigg, 2015; Campbell & Ward, 2017; Phillipson & Hammond, 2018; Dowlen et al., 2022; Fleetwood-Smith et al., 2022). These methods support and recognise alternative forms of communication, interaction and expression and thus can be considered essential when, for instance, exploring participation within traditional artistic practices which inherently involve multiple forms of expression, such as movement, gestures and actions (see for example: Zeilig et al., 2019).

In recent respective works by Thompson (2020) and Hatton (2021), they apply aesthetic, sensory lenses to practices within dementia care and unpick the intricacies around creative encounters to demonstrate intersections between care and creative practice. For example, Thompson (2020) explores an aesthetics of care through the connections made during participatory arts programmes, he illuminates the care and attentiveness within encounters in which value is placed within co-created moments rather than what the encounters 'produce'. This sensitive focus on the relational aspects of creative practice involves embracing multi-layered complexities around the co-creation of moments. Whilst Hatton (2021) draws our attention to the sensory environment as an important actant within creative encounters, she examines, for example, how bodies interact, respond to, and are mediated by the environments in which they are in. For instance, 'a movement exercise may stimulate an exchange of information via the sensation of the foot on the floor, whereas an exercise involving objects could initiate a different type of sensory encounter between the object and the fingertips' (2021: 75). Hatton (2021) claims that 'a sensory ecology for creative practice can draw attention to the broader range of creative possibilities available from and within a care space' (p. 77).

Nevertheless, it is important to acknowledge that participatory research methods that privilege the everyday are complex. Such approaches typically include multiple collaborators involving researchers, practitioners, people with dementia and those that surround them, and as such are resource heavy, time intensive and necessitate sensitivity, flexibility and reflexivity (Campbell et al., in press). To meet the needs of those involved, research funders increasingly advocate, if not necessitate, the involvement of patient and public contributors within the design, development and delivery of research. Yet such involvement can revolve around consultation with stakeholders, as opposed to practices which challenge asymmetrical power dynamics. Co-design and co-production models emphasise reciprocity and place the people involved at the centre of the research, yet there is a need to critically engage with such approaches particularly in relation to work with people with dementia (see for example: Lee, 2014; Hendriks et al., 2015) in order to ensure that their needs and wants are at the forefront of such research.

Developing research methods that attend to the everyday lives of people with dementia, connects with the move towards more-than-human and non-representational approaches to research. Although difficult to define, such approaches involve viewing the world as processual, dynamic and fluid. As Andrews et al. (2014) write 'non-representational theory does not see a world waiting to be examined, explained and theorised away. Its idea is that the world's living, ongoing and performative achievements should instead take centre stage including the many subtle, unspoken and often unintentional practices involved' (p. 165). Research underpinned by such concepts typically involves dynamic, improvisatory methods that attend to e.g. the social and material context of the research. For example, in Barron's (2021) research on the life-course of older adults they refer to the moment when the researcher produced a sweet from their pocket and this prompted the person they were researching with to recount a memory of an old sweet shop. It is these nuances and subtleties within the everyday that such approaches embrace and may be powerful in developing understanding around creativity in the lives of people with dementia.

Overall, this section has explored how we may begin to understand the uses of creativity in the everyday lives of people with dementia. By attending to the everyday, we can begin to move away from the ways in which arts and culture are 'sensationalised' in a dementia context. In Gray et al's (2018) work they suggest there are two commonplaces in the world of evaluating arts experiences in the context of dementia – '(1) it works and (2) this is hard to prove' (p. 776). Through our examination of methods that are used within this area, it is clear that framing the arts as interventions has led to a stagnation of research findings, with the same approaches often showing the same mixed findings. There needs to be further methodological innovation in this area to illuminate the everyday and centralise the voices and experiences of people with dementia.

Conclusion

This chapter has sought to unpack and challenge existing research and practice to examine what this area may look like moving forward. We have brought together narratives surrounding the value and perception of arts and culture in the lives of people with dementia and critically explored the ways in which the (bio)medical model of dementia continues to influence and limit our understanding of arts and culture in this area. We have explored these narratives through examining existing literature, sharing our own reflections and presenting selected examples from the media to explore the role of the arts in the lives of people with dementia.

Before concluding, we wish to reaffirm our position as two cisgender, white, non-disabled women, from middle-class backgrounds, who regularly engage with arts and culture. We work broadly within creative ageing and dementia research and are passionate about the importance of the arts within everyone's lives. The progression of the arts and dementia field is something that we are excited by, and our critical engagement does not seek to negate existing practice and research but build upon it. However, this is the first time we have engaged with a critical approach to understanding the value of the arts in the context of dementia – we have found it to be both illuminating and challenging on reflecting upon our own research practices. While critiquing the work of others, we are also aware of the pitfalls we may have fallen into working within this field and we aspire to take our reflections forward into future work as early career researchers.

To conclude, our examination of this area has led us to see a need for extending the trajectory of this area so that the arts can be reframed, reconsidered and reimagined in the lives of people with dementia. As discussed, this involves (1) continuing to critique the pervasive (bio)medical model of dementia that sees people with dementia treated as a homogenous group, (2) the development of innovative methodologies that foreground participatory, creative, sensory and embodied ways of knowing, (3) attending to the everyday lived experiences of people with dementia and (4) the repositioning of the arts as something far more meaningful than a magical 'elixir'. We do not claim that our reading of this area is without its limitations, and we acknowledge our respective personal/professional positions. However, we hope that our critical exploration may be useful in examining the future of arts and dementia and be useful in advocating for research/practice that embraces complexity and foregrounds creativity in the everyday lives of people with dementia.

References

Akhtar, F., Greenwood, N., Smith, R., & Richardson, A. (2017). Dementia cafés: recommendations from interviews with informal carers. *Working with Older People*.

All-Party Paliamentary Group on Arts, Health and Wellbeing (2017). *Creative Health: The Arts for Health and Wellbeing*. Retrieved from http://www.artshealthandwellbeing.org.uk/appg/inquiry

All-Party Parliamentary Group on Dementia. (2022). *Workforce Matters: Putting People Affected by Dementia at the Heart of Care*. Retrieved from https://www.alzheimers.org.uk/sites/default/files/2022-09/APPG%20on%20Dementia%20Workforce%20Matters%20Report%202022.pdf

Amanze, R. (2021). *Dementia, Music and Me*. Dementia, Diversity and the Arts. Retrieved from https://essexcdp.com/experience/dementia-diversity-and-the-arts/

Amponsem, S., Wolverson, E., & Clarke, C. (2022). The meaning and experience of hope by people living with dementia as expressed through poetry. *Dementia, 22*, 125–143. 14713012221137469.

Andrews, G. J., Chen, S., & Myers, S. (2014). The 'taking place' of health and wellbeing: Towards non-representational theory. *Social Science & Medicine, 108*, 210–222.

Baring Foundation. (2019). *Art and dementia in the UK South Asian Diaspora*. Retrieved from https://cdn.baringfoundation.org.uk/wp-content/uploads/BF_Art-dementia-in-UK-SA-Diaspora_Main-report_WEB.pdf

Barron, A. (2021). More-than-representational approaches to the life-course. *Social & Cultural Geography, 22*(5), 603–626.

Bartlett, R. (2015). Visualising dementia activism: Using the arts to communicate research findings. *Qualitative Research, 15*(6), 755–768.

Bartlett, R., & O'Connor, D. (2007). From personhood to citizenship: Broadening the lens for dementia practice and research. *Journal of Aging Studies, 21*(2), 107–118.

Basting, A. (2020). *Creative care: A revolutionary approach to dementia and elder care*. San Fransisco: HarperCollins.

Basting, A. D. (2006). Arts in dementia care: 'This is not the end … it's the end of this chapter.' *Generations, 30*(1), 16–20.

Basting, A., Towey, M., & Rose, E. (2016). *The Penelope project: An arts-based odyssey to change elder care*. Iowa City: University of Iowa Press.

Bellass, S., Balmer, A., May, V., Keady, J., Buse, C., Capstick, A., Burke, L., Bartlett, R., & Hodgson, J. (2019). Broadening the debate on creativity and dementia: A critical approach. *Dementia, 18*(7–8), 2799–2820.

Booth, R. (2021). Alzheimer's patients and hospital staff prescribed music in NHS trial. *The Guardian*. Retrieved from https://www.theguardian.com/science/2021/may/05/alzheimers-patients-and-hospital-staff-prescribed-music-in-nhs-trial#:~:text=A%20test%20among%20people%20with,and%20distress%20in%20some%20cases.

Bowell, S., & Bamford, S. M. (2018). What would life be–without a song or a dance what are we? *A Report from the Commission on Dementia and Music*. Retrieved from https://www.bl.uk/collection-items/what-would-life-be-without-a-song-or-dance-what-are-we-a-report-from-the-commission-on-dementia-and-music

Broome, E., Dening, T., & Schneider, J. (2020). Participatory arts in care settings: A multiple case study: Innovative practice. *Dementia, 19*(7), 2494–2503.

Buse, C. E., & Twigg, J. (2015). Clothing, embodied identity and dementia: maintaining the self through dress. *Age, Culture, Humanities 2*, 77–96.

Camic, P. M., Hulbert, S., & Kimmel, J. (2019). Museum object handling: A health-promoting community-based activity for dementia care. *Journal of Health Psychology, 24*(6), 787–798.

Campbell, S., Dowlen, R., & Fleetwood-Smith, R. (in press). Embracing complexity within creative approaches to dementia research: ethics, reflexivity, and research practices. *International Journal of Qualitative Methods*. doi:10.1177/16094069231165932

Campbell, S., & Ward, R. (2017). Video and observation data as a method to document practice and performances of gender in the dementia care-based hair salon: Practices and processes, In John Keady, Lars-Christer Hydén, Ann Johnson, Caroline Swarbrick (Eds.), *Social research methods in dementia studies* (pp. 96–118). Abingdon: Routledge.

Capstick, A., Chatwin, J., & Ludwin, K. (2015). Challenging representations of dementia in contemporary Western fiction film. In A. Swinnen and M. Schweda (Eds.), *Popularizing dementia: Public expressions and representations of forgetfulness.* Bielefeld: Transcript Verlag (Aging Studies, 6), 229–248.

Conroy, C. (2009). Disability: Creative tensions between drama, theatre and disability arts. *Research in Drama Education: The Journal of Applied Theatre and Performance, 14*(1), 1–14.

De Medeiros, K., & Basting, A. (2014). "Shall I compare thee to a dose of donepezil?": Cultural arts interventions in dementia care research. *The Gerontologist, 54*(3), 344–353.

De Nora, T. (2017). 'My Bonnie Dearie' In T. Stickley & S. Clift (Eds.), *Arts, health and wellbeing: A theoretical inquiry for practice.* Newcastle upon Tyne: Cambridge Scholars Publisher.

Dodd, D. (2018). How to harness music to fight dementia. *Financial Times.* Retreived from https://www.ft.com/content/62f912b0-100a-11e8-8cb6-b9ccc4c4dbbb

Dowlen, R., & Keady, J. (forthcoming). Open University Press. In K. Gray, C. Russell, & J. Twigg (Eds.), *Considering leisure in the context of dementia.* London: Open University Press

Dowlen, R., Keady, J., Milligan, C., Swarbrick, C., Ponsillo, N., Geddes, L., & Riley, B. (2022). In the moment with music: An exploration of the embodied and sensory experiences of people living with dementia during improvised music-making. *Ageing & Society, 42*(11), 2642–2664.

Dowson, B., Atkinson, R., Barnes, J., Barone, C., Cutts, N., Donnebaum, E., Hung Hsu, M., Lo Coco, I., John, G., & Meadows, G. (2021). Digital approaches to music-making for people with dementia in response to the COVID-19 pandemic: current practice and recommendations. *Frontiers in Psychology, 12*, 625258.

Dupuis, S. L., Kontos, P., Mitchell, G., Jonas-Simpson, C., & Gray, J. (2016). Re-claiming citizenship through the arts. *Dementia, 15*(3), 358–380.

European Union Agency for Fundamental Rights. (2017). *Fundamental Rights Report 2017.* Retrieved from https://fra.europa.eu/sites/default/files/fra_uploads/fra-2017-fundamental-rights-report-2017_en.pdf

Fleetwood-Smith, R. (2020). *Exploring the significance of clothing to people with dementia using sensory ethnography.* London: University of West London.

Fleetwood-Smith, R., Tischler, V., & Robson, D. (2022). Using creative, sensory and embodied research methods when working with people with dementia: A method story. *Arts & Health, 14*(3), 263–279.

Fletcher, J. R. (2021). Unethical governance: Capacity legislation and the exclusion of people diagnosed with dementias from research. *Research Ethics, 17*(3), 298–308.

Gray, K., Evans, S. C., Griffiths, A., & Schneider, J. (2018). Critical reflections on methodological challenge in arts and dementia evaluation and research. *Dementia, 17*(6), 775–784.

Hatton, N. (2021). A Relational Approach to Dementia Care. In Nicky Hatton (Ed.), *Performance and Dementia* (pp. 63–87). Cham: Springer.

Hendriks, N., Slegers, K., & Duysburgh, P. (2015). Codesign with people living with cognitive or sensory impairments: A case for method stories and uniqueness. *CoDesign, 11*(1), 70–82.

James, I. A., & Jackman, L. (2017). *Understanding behaviour in dementia that challenges: A guide to assessment and treatment.* London: Jessica Kingsley Publishers.

Keady, J. D., Campbell, S., Clark, A., Dowlen, R., Elvish, R., Jones, L., Kindell, J., Swarbrick, C., & Williams, S. (2022). Re-thinking and re-positioning 'being in the moment' within a continuum of moments: Introducing a new conceptual framework for dementia studies. *Ageing & Society*, *42*(3), 681–702.

Kinsey, D., Lang, I., Orr, N., Anderson, R., & Parker, D. (2021). The impact of including carers in museum programmes for people with dementia: a realist review. *Arts & Health*, *13*(1), 1–19.

Kontos, P. C. (2004). Ethnographic reflections on selfhood, embodiment and Alzheimer's disease. *Ageing & Society*, *24*(6), 829–849.

Kontos, P. C. (2005). Embodied selfhood in Alzheimer's disease: Rethinking person-centred care. *Dementia*, *4*(4), 553–570.

Kontos, P., Grigorovich, A., & Colobong, R. (2020). Towards a critical understanding of creativity and dementia: new directions for practice change. *International Practice Development Journal*, *10*, 1–13.

Kontos, P., Miller, K. L., & Kontos, A. P. (2017). Relational citizenship: Supporting embodied selfhood and relationality in dementia care. *Sociology of Health & Illness*, *39*(2), 182–198.

Lee, J.-J. (2014). The true benefits of designing design methods. *Artifact: Journal of Design Practice*, *3*(2), 5.1–5.12.

Leighton, F. (2009). Accountability: the ethics of devising a practice-as-research performance with learning-disabled practitioners. *RiDE: The Journal of Applied Theatre and Performance*, *14*(1), 97–113.

Letrondo, P. A., Ashley, S. A., Flinn, A., Burton, A., Kador, T., & Mukadam, N. (2022). Systematic review of arts and culture-based interventions for people living with dementia and their caregivers. *Ageing Research Reviews*, 101793, 1–9

Macleod, F., Storey, L., Rushe, T., & McLaughlin, K. (2021). Towards an increased understanding of reminiscence therapy for people with dementia: A narrative analysis. *Dementia*, *20*(4), 1375–1407.

Mak, H. W., Coulter, R., & Fancourt, D. (2020). Patterns of social inequality in arts and cultural participation: Findings from a nationally representative sample of adults living in the United Kingdom of Great Britain and Northern Ireland. *Public Health Panorama: Journal of the WHO Regional Office for Europe= Panorama obshchestvennogo zdravookhraneniia*, *6*(1), 55.

Moisse, K. (2012). Alzheimer's Disease: Music Brings Patients 'Back to Life'. *ABC News*. Retrieved from https://abcnews.go.com/Health/AlzheimersCommunity/alzheimers-disease-music-brings-patients-back-life/story?id=16117602

Nedlund, A.-C., Bartlett, R., & Clarke, C. (2019). *Everyday citizenship and people with dementia*. Edinburgh: Dunedin Academic Press Ltd.

Phillipson, L., & Hammond, A. (2018). More than talking: A scoping review of innovative approaches to qualitative research involving people with dementia. *International Journal of Qualitative Methods*, *17*(1), 1609406918782784.

Shakespeare, T., Zeilig, H., & Mittler, P. (2019). Rights in mind: Thinking differently about dementia and disability. *Dementia*, *18*(3), 1075–1088.

Skyes, P. (2022). Doing it Right with Pandora Sykes In *What we get wrong about dementia with Wendy Mitchell*. Retrieved from https://doingitright.podbean.com/e/what-we-get-wrong-about-dementia-with-wendy-mitchell/

Swaffer, K. (2016). Co-production and engagement of people with dementia: The issue of ethics and creative or intellectual copyright. *Dementia*, *15*, 1319–1325.

Tapson, C., Noble, D., Daykin, N., & Walters, D. (2018). *Live Music in Care: The impact of music interventions for people living and working in care home settings.* Retrieved from https://achoirineverycarehome.files.wordpress.com/2018/11/live-music-in-care.pdf

The Unfurlings. (n.d.). *The Unfurlings project.* Retrieved from https://theunfurlings.org.uk/

Thompson, J. (2020). Towards an aesthetics of care. In Amanda Stuart Fisher, James Thompson (Eds.), *Performing care* (pp. 36–48). Manchester: Manchester University Press.

Tsekleves, E., & Keady, J. (2021). *Design for people living with dementia: Interactions and innovations.* Routledge.

UK Music & Music for Dementia. (2022). *Power of Music: A plan for harnessing music to improve our health, wellbeing and communities.* Retrieved from https://musicfordementia.org.uk/wp-content/uploads/2022/04/Power-of-Music-Report.pdf

van der Byl Williams, M., & Zeilig, H. (2022). Broadening and deepening the understanding of agency in dementia. *Medical Humanities, 49,* 38–47.

Van der Steen, J. T., Smaling, H. J., Van der Wouden, J. C., Bruinsma, M. S., Scholten, R. J., & Vink, A. C. (2018). Music-based therapeutic interventions for people with dementia. *Cochrane Database of Systematic Reviews* (7).

Zeilig, H., Killick, J., & Fox, C. (2014). The participative arts for people living with a dementia: a critical review. *International Journal of Ageing and Later Life, 9*(1), 7–34.

Zeilig, H., Tischler, V., van der Byl Williams, M., West, J., & Strohmaier, S. (2019). Co-creativity, well-being and agency: A case study analysis of a co-creative arts group for people with dementia. *Journal of Aging Studies, 49,* 16–24.

Part V
Politics

11 Human rights and dementia

A 'Socratic dialogue'

Toby Williamson and Nick Jenkins

Prologue

This chapter is based on an exchange of academic letters between Williamson and Jenkins that took place between March and August 2022. Extracts from these letters have been edited and re-ordered in order to create a *Socratic Dialogue* between the two authors, on the contribution that *Human Rights Based Approaches* (HRBA) have made to the field of dementia studies. Toby Williamson is an independent health- and social-care consultant and works in dementia research, education, policy and service development. For ten years he was *Head of Later Life* at the Mental Health Foundation, a UK social research and development charity where he led a number of projects focusing on people's lived experiences of dementia and issues of equality, diversity and inclusion (EDI). Nicholas Jenkins is a *Senior Lecturer in Sociology & Social Policy* at the University of the West of Scotland. He has worked in the field of dementia research and activism since 2012, and currently co-convenes the Multispecies Dementia International Research Network; an academic network dedicated to exploring more-than-human approaches to dementia (https://multispeciesdementia.org/).

As will become clear, Williamson and Jenkins hold differing views on the contributions that HRBA have made, and can make, to advancing dementia policy and practice. By engaging with each other in constructive dialogue, and *Slow* scholarship (Berg and Seeber, 2016) they strived to achieve a position of mutual understanding and, through doing so, identify potential areas for future thinking, discussion and research.

The discussion

Introductions

Williamson: I would like to describe the background to how human rights have become a significant feature in the lives of people living with dementia, family and friends who support them, as well as policy and practice for dementia care more widely. I will outline some of the evidence which I believe indicates that human rights-based approaches (HRBA) have brought benefits to both theory and practice

DOI: 10.4324/9781003290353-17

in dementia care. My examples will tend to be UK-focused but they reflect international thinking and trends. The move towards conceptualising dementia in terms of rights and the social model of disability has real potential to challenge negative perceptions of the condition, as well as institutionalised, discriminatory or abusive practice (personal experiences of which are discussed by Mason and colleagues and the Scottish Dementia Alumni in Chapters 3 and 12, respectively). In our discussion, I will outline some of the evidence which I believe indicates the benefits that HRBA have brought. However, I am aware that you may have different views and I therefore look forward to a dialogue between the two of us.

Jenkins: It is a pleasure to engage in a discussion with you around the contribution that human rights-based approaches (HRBA) have made to our understandings of dementia. I have followed your work with great interest, and how you have sought to apply social perspectives on disability to the field of dementia; as outlined, for example, in Williamson (2015a,b). Your consideration of how socio-legal frameworks such as the *Human Rights Act* 1998, the *Equality Act* 2010 and the *Care Act 2014* may enable people living with dementia to exercise their human rights across both macro- and micro levels of society is highly engaging and deeply thought provoking. I hope to learn a lot from you through this exchange.

Williamson: Thank you for those words. I am not so familiar with your work but I suspect (and hope) that I am also about to learn much from you. In actual fact, ten years ago, in 2012 when I had been active in the field of dementia for some time, the relevance of human rights was virtually nowhere on my agenda. But the penny began to drop around that time when I heard a prominent campaigner living with dementia, Chris Roberts, describe his dementia as a disability. This put me on a journey, via an outstanding conference presentation by Gráinne McGettrick (then Research and Policy Manager at the Alzheimer Society of Ireland) about the HRBA in relation to dementia, to leading on a project resulting in the publication of *Dementia, Rights and the Social Model of Disability* (Mental Health Foundation, 2015). This was certainly not the first time that dementia had been conceptualised in terms of human rights, and as a disability (Bartlett, 2000; Gwilliam & Gilliard, 1996) but it did attract a lot of interest and helped build a wider narrative and awareness.

Prior to the 2015 report, human rights in relation to dementia had mainly been concerned with issues to do with the rights to liberty, and the right to privacy and family life (Article 5 and Article 8 of the *European Convention on Human Rights*, which underpins the UK's *Human Rights Act*). These were clearly important for health and social care practitioners to understand in order to ensure that people with dementia were not unduly restricted when living in care homes for example, and publications tended to focus on these issues. But issues such as deprivations of liberty were still largely based on a *biopsychosocial*[1] model of dementia, focused on the individual. Within this model, the historic dominance of the 'biomedical' over the 'psychosocial' (see Chapter 1 by Fletcher) and the slow process of prioritising dementia in policy terms and policy implementation in the UK for example,[2] contributed much to the damaging way in which dementia was perceived and responded to, reflected in the stigma, discrimination and poor quality of service that many people affected by dementia had experienced.[3]

Leaving aside my journey, the growing collective voice of people with dementia seeking to raise awareness and change attitudes and services through networks such as the *Dementia Engagement and Empowerment Project* (DEEP),[4] (members of which have authored Chapter 3), and the *Dementia Alliance International* (DAI),[5] helped, somewhat ironically, by the development of 'dementia friendly communities' over the last ten years, have been important in giving human rights a broader focus in policy and practice terms.[6] This is reflected in the 2015 report and other more recent publications, including those by people with other disabilities and dementia (Shakespeare et al., 2019). Instead of focusing on the pathology of dementia as the problem, these developments considered dementia much more in terms of social inclusion, citizenship and equalities. This involved using a fairly loose definition of the social model of disability (originally developed by people with disabilities), requiring society to adapt to support people with dementia, rather than a biopsychosocial model focused mainly on 'fixing' the individual but also taking into account people's lived experience of their dementia and the distress this could sometimes cause them. This has not only been important in reframing dementia in a more positive way, but it has also raised awareness of the clear link with human rights frameworks such as the *United Nations Convention on the Rights of Persons with Disabilities* (UN-CRPD) which includes positive rights (e.g. access to services, being able to participate in civic life), and the UK's *Equality Act* 2010, both of which are both based on the social model of disability. Many of these ideas were explored and expanded upon in a book I co-authored, *The Dementia Manifesto* (Hughes & Williamson, 2019).

The challenge

Jenkins: Many thanks for establishing our discussion on the role of human rights based approaches (HRBA) in dementia. I found this very thought-provoking, and it has helped me to explore my own thinking in this area. As you know, my own perspective on HRBA in dementia differs somewhat from yours. As a post-humanist (a theoretical standpoint outlined by Lotherington in Chapter 6), multi-species researcher, I am deeply sceptical of the value that *human* rights-based discourses bring to dementia, as well as the potential for such frameworks to bring about radical change. Whilst, as you highlight, HRBA in dementia tends to be associated with the rise of 'the social model of disability' in reality, it has a much older and a much more chequered history than this. As the socio-legal scholar D'Souza (2018) highlights, the rise of human rights in both law and philosophy can be traced back to the *European Enlightenment* (1685–1815) where the language of rights played a central role in legitimating projects of colonialism and the forced displacement of indigenous populations in the centuries that followed. As such, it was actually during the late 1700s that the first attempts were made to assert the fundamental humanity, and inalienable human rights of people affected by dementia, by the pioneers of *Moral Treatment*, such as Philippe Pinel (1745–1826) in France, and William Tuke (1732–1822) in the UK. Arguably, their assertions that members of the 'insane' community, including people with dementia ('abolition of the thinking faculty') were far more radical then (see Fletcher on Pinel in Chapter 1), compared with our contemporary attempts to recognise the human rights of people with dementia. Why, then, two hundred years later, has so little changed? I believe it is because HRBA in dementia suffer from an inescapable paradox, which is that by seeking to highlight the ways in which people with dementia are people 'first' (Kitwood 1997) – and therefore worthy of the exceptional moral and legal considerations that *Personhood* affords – they inadvertently re-enforce the very logic of human exceptionalism[7] which they seek to resist. As posthumanists such as Cary Wolfe (2003) and Rosi Braidotti (2013) highlight, there are close historical connections between human exceptionalism, *speciesism*[8] and more human-centred forms of oppression, including, ableism, ethnocentrism, sexism and racism. To my mind, as long as HRBA in dementia remains rooted in conventional (i.e. liberal humanist) understandings of what it means to be human, such as those espoused by Kitwood (1997), they will never be able to escape this self-defeating form of logic.

Williamson: I'm not sure I accept the assertion that HRBA in conjunction with Kitwood's notion of personhood reinforce all the human-centred forms of oppression you describe. I'm not clear what evidence there is to support this argument. I do accept that some aspects of 'personhood' are challenged by current notions of EDI, and I am not trying to deny the existence of exceptionalism and speciesism. However, there are tools that can be used to develop HRBA which explicitly challenge inequalities, such as the PANEL principles as used in Scotland.[9] Furthermore, jettisoning the principles of person-centred care that underpins personhood, risks undermining the good practice in dementia care that has been developed over the last 20 years.

Space does not permit me to explore the issues you raise about HRBA and its relation to historical knowledge-power structures, but I agree with you that HRBA can become a smokescreen used by those in power for inaction or for ulterior motives. But when people with dementia articulate rights in progressive ways it's important to respect their agency and support them.

However, the points you make raise serious questions about whether the benefits of HRBA that I described are outweighed by both practical and theoretical drawbacks to the approach. Would you conclude that HRBA is inherently flawed, even retrogressive, or at best, has resulted in a policy and practice cul-de-sac and can make no further progress?

Before you answer that question, perhaps it's also worth emphasising, though not necessarily framed in terms of human rights the succession of reports and news items about the poor quality of care provided to people with dementia, which can easily be reconceptualised as a violation of their rights. For example, a 2014 report about hospitals and care homes in England stated:

> It is likely that someone living with dementia will experience poor care at some point while living in a care home or being treated in hospital.
>
> (Care Quality Commission, 2014, p. 3)

This strikes me as unacceptable; the rights to health and social care that a person with dementia has should not be caveated in this way.

More recently the COVID-19 pandemic demonstrated how the most fundamental human right – the right to life – could in effect be suspended for people with dementia in order notionally to protect the lives of others, although the slogan in the UK of 'protect the NHS' rather suggested an institution was the priority, not people. At the beginning of the pandemic the lack of availability of PPE equipment in care homes and hospital discharge decisions that led to many people with dementia, often with suspected COVID-19, being discharged from hospital directly to care homes (irrespective of whether it was in their legally defined 'best interests') helped dementia to become the most common pre-morbid condition for people who died of COVID-19 (CTJ, 2022). For those that lived, further human rights violations occurred in terms of being denied access to health care or to have meaningful contact with family or friends if they lived in care homes (Suárez-González et al., 2020). To add insult to injury, 12 months into the pandemic, dementia was still not named as a condition which the UK government deemed worthy of including in their list of conditions which made people clinically vulnerable to the virus.[10]

Jenkins: I do not see HRBA as being either retrogressive or without merit. As you rightly state, HRBA has led to tangible gains for many people living with progressive neurocognitive conditions; gains which, arguably, would not have been made had dementia policy and practice remained rooted in the conventional biopsychosocial understandings. I see HRBA as a pragmatically useful framework for putting dementia policy and practice on a path towards more progressive and less oppressive forms of treatment. However, I remain sceptical about the potential of HRBA to bring about *radical* change. Following critical scholars such as Wolfe (2003; 2010), Haraway (2008; 2016) and Barad (2007), I believe that there *is* a more radical ethical, ontological and epistemological project through which social hierarchies, founded upon human exceptionalism, can be de-stabilised. HRBA, I fear, risk obscuring that project and thus preventing us from *thinking otherwise* about dementia. Whilst recent formulations have sought to recast and broaden the criteria upon which human rights are granted, this does little to challenge the underlying *episteme* of exceptionalism upon which much discrimination and oppression has historically been based (Braidotti, 2013; Foucault, 1966/2002). In contrast, from the disability field, there is an emerging body of work amongst activists, scholars and artists that identifies affinities and connection with what Abrams (1996) refers to as the '*more-than-human world*' – an animist realm of sensuous experience upon which our very subjectivity (and humanity) depends, yet which the ideology of human exceptionalism has come to demarcate as inanimate and ontologically distinct from human experience. A very poignant example of this is the work of Finnish artist and disability activist Jenni-Juulia Wallinheimo-Heimonen, whose recent work explores human-animal relations within disability art (see, for example, *Authority Experience* and *the Battle of Scarcity of Resource*). Within academia, research at the intersections of critical disability studies and critical animal studies is increasingly exploring connections between ableism and speciesism, which I highlighted earlier, as mutually re-enforcing systems of oppression. Such academic coalitions, whilst far from being without tension or controversy, have potential to inject new forms of energy and lead to new forms of mobilisation because they help disrupt, destabilise and reconfigure what it means to *Be* human'. As Martino and Lindsay (2020, pp. 2–3) state:

> *Disabled people bring rich perspectives around interdependence, creative ways of mobilising, and making space for non-normative ways of voicing lived experience. At the same time, critical animal studies can contribute to disability studies scholarship and activism through its extensive work on advocating for the "voiceless" through a holistic approach, which considers all beings and environments, through our social relationships and unavoidably interdependent existences.*

Williamson: I agree that taking a wider perspective is important in this discussion. There is evidence of narratives, as well as real life events, that link disability activism, dementia, rights-based approaches, and constructing wider alliances, that could develop into the collaborations you suggest. A cursory scan of the literature reveals some interesting studies linking air pollution and temperature change with the prevalence of dementia (Guzmán et al., 2022; Wei, 2019). McShane (2018) draws an analogy between the need to adapt one's love for a family member whose behaviour has become strange and unpredictable as a result of dementia, and the need to adapt our love and concern for the natural world as it is affected by climate change. As one might expect there is much more literature exploring the effect of climate change on people with disabilities, too much to list here. However, I was particularly interested in a number of articles that critiqued a discourse about people with disabilities as being portrayed solely as victims of climate change, and tried instead to position them as potential agents of change, linking disability rights with activism around climate change and power imbalances more widely (e.g. Stein and Stein, 2022; Watts Belser, 2020). Many people with dementia (and family carers) are now consciously exercising their agency on numerous issues, as evidenced through networks such as DEEP and the DAI. This has included a focus on rights as well as recognising common ground with other disability groups, such as successfully campaigning alongside autism pressure groups in the UK to get 'hidden' disabilities properly recognised as grounds for being entitled to blue badge disabled parking permits (Alzheimer's Society, 2019; Press Association, 2018).

The 'dementia friendly community' movement, though not always HRBA-focused, partly reflects a social model of disability as well as what one could describe as 'entanglements' (Barad, 2007) with all sorts of organisations that hitherto had no associations with dementia, such as shops and businesses, public transport, and the arts, culture and heritage sectors (McGettrick and Williamson, 2015; Rahman and Swaffer, 2018; Shannon et al., 2019; Williamson, 2016). Links have also been made between dementia and the natural environment which, though not overtly about climate change, have the potential to go in the direction you suggest (Hendriks et al., 2016; Mapes et al., 2016). Explorations of the different realities and 'truths' that people with dementia may experience such as time-shifting back into their past lives can, as you say, 'disrupt, destabilise and reconfigure what it means to *Be* human' (Kirtley and Williamson, 2016; Hughes and Williamson, 2019). All these examples contain elements of rights-based approaches, some more loosely than others, but they would not have occurred if dementia remained rooted in a conventional biopsychosocial model'.

Jenkins: Indeed. Dementia studies and dementia activism has much to offer these new terrains, yet the field has been slow to engage with these areas of critical inquiry. Dementia fundamentally challenges us to re-think our understandings of subjectivity, agency, personhood and self-hood in ways that ripple *beyond* the 'human', as constructed within liberal humanist discourse, which in turn create important opportuni-ties for re-framing our relations in the *more than human world*.

Williamson: Though perhaps still somewhat anthropocentric, these narra-tives seem to describe potential vehicles for enabling HRBA to be broader and more inclusive, perhaps dropping the 'H' to allow the 'R' to include the rights of other sentient beings and natural phe-nomena, and maybe therefore addressing some of the critiques you make of HRBA?

Jenkins: Whilst I see the logic of this and the potential for pragmatic gains, I re-main sceptical about the emancipatory potential of making hierarchical ethical-legal frameworks (such as HRBA) more inclusive. Rather than 'dropping the 'H'', I wonder if we need to *reconfigure* the H; through, for example, greater acknowledgement that we only *become* human through our relations with (non-human) life. The human body does not consist exclusively of human cells, neither has human DNA evolved in isolation from other species (see: Gilbert, Sapp & Tauber, 2012; Margulis, 1970). The human body is *symbiotic* as opposed to *autopo-etic*, so rather than viewing the human as an essentialised, pre-social and exceptional form of Being, understanding how we *become* human through our entanglements with other species can help us cultivate new ways of understanding not only personhood in dementia, but the lived experience of dementia itself. Similarly, rather than 'allowing the 'R' to include the rights of other sentient beings ...' I wonder if we would be better to move *beyond* the language of rights, *towards* the language of '*response-ability*'. Response-ability, in this context, is not meant as the natural corollary of rights. Rather, it is the cultivation of the capacity to respond, with others, for the worlds that we are *for* (Haraway, 2016). Working together, within and across species, for the worlds we wish to being into being may lead to 'opening up possibilities for different kinds of responses' (Schrader, 2010, p. 299) in dementia in ways that are difficult to fully conceptualise just now, as long as we remain *shack-led* (Latimer, 2014) to the ideology of human exceptionalism. So my question to you, is how can we explore such *response-ability* in demen-tia in ways that continue to position the experiences, realities, truths and choices of people living dementia at the centre and which continue to uphold and support the agency of those who have historically been disempowered through oppressive, ableist forms of discourse?

Williamson: I think there are two ways the concept of *response-ability* could be explored, which are not mutually exclusive and can be in dialogue with each other. Firstly, there could be a continuation of what we have been doing here i.e. a theoretical discussion that considers the interplay of all the elements you describe, as well as external factors (the political, cultural and socio-economic environment, etc.) which will have a bearing on that. But secondly, and what is much more challenging, is to actually find ways of doing that exploration in ways that are inclusive and meaningful for people with lived experience of dementia, together with other disability activists, climate change campaigners, and others challenging things like speciesism. Both ways of exploring 'response-ability' are demanding activities and I'm sure you would agree that the second one poses a number of practical challenges. Not least of these is to ensure that the language we use and the way issues are explored are accessible for people affected by dementia. When I was involved in developing the ideas behind *Dementia, Rights and the Social Model of Disability* (Mental Health Foundation 2015) a person with dementia advising on the project expressed concern because he felt that being called 'disabled' was negatively labelling him. I suspect this view may still be quite common, so supporting people with dementia to make the link with disability, let alone speciesism and human exceptionalism, remains a necessary but major challenge.

Furthermore, great care has to be taken if links are drawn between the different realities and truths that people with dementia may experience and your desire to 'disrupt, destabilise and reconfigure what it means to *Be* human'. It's not difficult to see how this could be subverted into something extremely reactionary and dangerous by relegating people with dementia to a 'sub-human' category, in the way people with learning disabilities and mental health problems, Jews and other minority groups were treated with devastating consequences by the Nazis.

Jenkins: You raise a really important point, when you say that doing *response-ability* in dementia needs to be enacted in ways that are inclusive and meaningful to people living with neurocognitive conditions - I could not agree more! Key to practicing response-ability, to my mind, is generating a community that, through its shared explorations, identity and endeavours is capable of increasing our shared capacity to respond to the challenges, and opportunities, that dementia presents. Cultivating more 'mutant' approaches to subjectivity, as Braidotti (2013) suggests, can only be done *with* people with lived experiences of neurocognitive disorders. Drawing on posthuman theory, Quinn and Blandon (2020) offer us '*beyond words*' and, potentially, beyond HRBA-based methodologies, for doing just that.

You are absolutely right that attempts to move *beyond* the language of (human) rights need to be vigilant to reactionary efforts to subvert or otherwise misrepresent such a project. Understanding the ways in which human subjectivity is produced through our relations with more than human life cannot, and should *never* be, portrayed as an attempt to relegate those living with neurocognitive conditions, or any other form of impairment for that matter, to the status of 'sub-human'. Indeed, one of the main motivators for going beyond HRBA approaches is precisely to avoid unhelpful and epistemologically unstable bifurcations between human and non-human through which liminal statuses such as 'sub-human' are made possible. Understanding the ways in which we (all of us) *become* human, ipso-facto, involves considering humanity's relations with the non-human at both the conceptual and material levels. This does not diminish our humanity. On the contrary, it involves attending to the ways in which our relations with the more-than-human contribute to our becoming <u>as</u> human beings'.

The paths ahead

Williamson: I think we are moving towards a degree of consensus. If some kind of theoretical and practical alliance is going to be built that links dementia, climate change, and interspecies relations I think there are two approaches that could be taken to help try and ensure it's accessible and meaningful for people affected by dementia. The first way uses the language of rights to make the link between dementia and the natural world. I've already given some examples of this but the move to designate rivers as living beings and thereby have legal 'personhood' with their own rights which can be represented in law, in order to protect them, is one such example (Magallanes, 2018; O'Donnell, 2020; O'Donnell and Talbot-Jones, 2018; Pecharroman, 2018). Rights of nature are most commonly advocated for by indigenous people in post-colonial countries where they are striving to protect traditional land and the conceptualisation of rights therefore draws upon non-Western legal traditions and it is not without its own controversies (O'Donnell, 2020). Nevertheless, it provides an accessible entry point for discussion about the links between human rights and the natural environment. The *Equality Act* reminds us that riverside walks should be accessible to people with cognitive impairments as well as physical impairments; what better way to make the links between rights, nature, dementia and disability than by strolling with people affected by dementia and talking about this alongside a meandering river?

The second approach focuses on notions of inequality, one of which clearly exists where you've described the status of how humans are viewed compared to other sentient beings and the planet, more generally. In recent years there has been much greater interest shown in how wider inequalities in society are replicated or exaggerated for people affected by dementia, according to characteristics of age, gender, race and ethnicity, sexual orientation, disability and socio-economic status (Voluntary Organisations Disabilities Group, 2016). 'Oh, we are back to rights-based thinking' you might say. Well, yes, we are, but I would argue that an important reason why there is still no cure for dementia, and treatments are of limited effectiveness is because of inequalities. Two factors in dementia not being deemed to be a priority for so long, compared to cancer for example, I believe were endemic ageism (dementia, seen wrongly, only as condition of old age) and sexism (women are much more likely to be affected by dementia directly, or indirectly as carers). But I actually want to suggest that the impact of inequalities go further than this and start making links with the work of people like Kate Pickett and Richard Wilkinson on inequalities issues such as life expectancy (Wilkinson and Pickett, 2010). For example, we know that while the risk of developing dementia is higher among lower income groups, the prevalence is higher among more affluent groups, largely because the latter live longer which is linked with the social and economic advantages they enjoy (Voluntary Organisations Disabilities Group, 2016). And while dementia is a growing challenge globally, inequalities between countries are reflected in the capacity of their health and social care systems to respond to the challenge posed by the condition.

Obviously there is a much bigger debate about the causes of inequalities but there is plenty of evidence to show that a key driver for inequality is the socio-economic system we live in, capitalism put bluntly, which is also a driver for global warming, environmental destruction and species' extinction. So perhaps inequality provides another accessible link between dementia, rights and the issues you raise. There is a certain irony here, that while so much attention and effort is expended on trying to save the four-billion-year old planet earth, far less attention is paid to a socio-economic system that has only become dominant in the last 500 years. As the cultural theorist, Mark Fisher, said, 'it's easier to imagine the end of the world than the end of capitalism' (Fisher, 2009). Can we start enabling people affected by dementia to imagine being part of a world that supports them to live well with dementia as full and equal citizens on a planet that also respects the rights of other sentient beings and the natural environment. A planet which is not dominated by a socio-economic system that is destroying the earth, and only respects 'rights' based on the profit motive, materialism and gross inequalities in wealth?

Jenkins: The two pathways you present for forming connections between HRBA and the '*post*' approaches to dementia are very interesting. I must admit to leaning more towards the second strategy. Whilst, I agree, presenting access to nature and natural environments in terms of *rights* can lead to pragmatic gains, I find myself returning to the questions of: (a) Whose responsibility is it to ensure such rights are upheld? Is it, for example, the responsibility of States, supra-national organisations, or individuals? (b) What happens when those rights are violated, as they all-too-often are? Your second pathway, entangling social justice and environmental justice through the lens of *inequality*, to my mind, offers us a more promising opportunities for establishing new, flexible forms of coalition. As you say, drawing on Fisher (2009), our ability to imagine a world beyond capitalism is highly constrained. This is where *tentacular thinking*,[11] *with* the more-than-human in mind, may offer us new directions. In the *Mushroom at the End of the World*, for example, Tsing (2015) argues that the life of a rare and highly sought-after form of fungi, the *Matsutake*, can offer humans important insights through which we can cultivate new strategies for living well on an increasingly precarious planet, characterised by increasing levels of capitalist-fuelled environmental degradation. Exploring the ability of the *Matsutake* mushroom to thrive in the landscapes of capitalist ruin, far from being an exercise in despair, Tsing argues, can provide humans with new sources of optimism.

To live with dementia is, I believe, to live at the margins of the capitalist *logos*. As Wilkie (2015) highlights, whilst those at the margins are often exposed to oppression, ridicule, exclusion and tarnish, the margins are also places where innovation and experimentation thrive. With unique insights and experiences, people with dementia may well be some of the best placed to imagine life beyond our current capitalist logos. Truly leaning-in and attending to such sensuous experience, may (I truly hope) help reveal new ways of imagining life and humanity that go beyond human exceptionalist frames of reference.

Williamson: This dialogue has been immensely valuable and I'm very grateful because so many points you raise have challenged my thinking and enabled me to consider rights and dementia from a new perspective. It's absolutely right to raise awareness of the epistemological foundations of HRBA which have led to exceptionalism, discrimination and oppression. Yet, to re-emphasise my earlier point, unless one argues that people with dementia are 'victims' of 'false consciousness' which therefore deprives them of agency (and a traditional disease model of dementia is very good at doing that in any case), HRBA where people with dementia have been pro-active, have brought <u>some</u> tangible benefits for <u>some</u> people affected by dementia. I think this is a reminder of what we have attempted in this dialogue, to try and straddle two tasks simultaneously. Firstly, critical thinking about current and developing concepts in dementia, and secondly sharing evidence about what could make a radical and progressive practical difference to people affected by the condition. Perhaps our dialogue has found some common ground between HRBA and multi-species, post-humanist approaches which enable both to evolve in a way that will be beneficial, though not exclusively, to people affected by dementia.

Jenkins: Yes, I think one area we can agree on is that, whilst we need to be mindful of their historical origins and epistemological assumptions, human rights-based approaches have brought *some* tangible benefits to *some* people affected by dementia. Rights-based thinking has, in recent years, led to a number of oppressive practices being challenged (e.g. inappropriate prescribing of anti-psychotic medications) and to practical frameworks capable of developing more progressive approaches to dementia care, such as the *PANEL* framework.[12] Simultaneously thinking critically *with* and *about* human rights is, as you say, a tricky endeavour. Yet doing so helps us avoid the trap of thinking that any single approach – be it HRBA, multi-speciesism or post-humanist –, presents us with a panacea capable of addressing and resolving all instances of oppression and discrimination in dementia. It is for this reason, perhaps, that dialogues such as ours, where advocates and sceptics can engage in constructive and mutually supportive conversations with each other, are so important.

Notes

1 The biopsychosocial model is a conceptual and practical framework widely used to understand and treat long term health conditions. First conceptualised by George Engel in 1977, it views health conditions as being combinations of the pathological, psychological and socio-environmental factors affecting the individual and a multi-disciplinary approach to care and treatment that can address all these factors is therefore required (Engel, 1977).

2 Successive UK Labour governments between 1997 and 2010 published a number of national health strategies, including mental health (1999), coronary heart disease (2000), learning disabilities (2001), diabetes (2003) and long-term health conditions (2005). Dementia was referred to in the strategy for older people's health, published in 2001 but only had five pages specifically devoted to it; the strategy had 202 pages. The first national dementia strategy was published in 2009 (Department of Health, 2009).

3 See: National Audit Office (2007); National Audit Office (2013).

4 https://www.dementiavoices.org.uk/

5 https://www.dementiaallianceinternational.org/

6 The irony of dementia friendly communities (DFCs) helping to support HRBA is that in England they were a policy initiative led by a Conservative-led coalition government and can be seen as the state abdicating statutory responsibility for the provision of care, while using an approach that owes far more to a social model of disability for dementia than more traditional biomedical models. In some other European countries, DFCs were more closely aligned with rights-based approaches (see Williamson, 2014).

7 Human exceptionalism refers to the ontological belief that humans possess exceptional characteristics and attributes (such as the capacity for language) which, in turn, make humans deserving of superior moral status and enhanced legal protections.

8 Speciesism refers to prejudice in favour of members of one's own species and against members of other species. It was first proposed by the psychologist Richard D. Ryder and subsequently popularised by the animal liberationist Peter Singer during the 1970s.

9 https://www.scottishhumanrights.com/projects-and-programmes/human-rights-based-approach/

10 Dementia was eventually added to this list.

11 Tentacular thinking is an approach advocated by Donna Haraway (2016). It stems from the Latin *tentare*, which amongst others, evokes attempts to *try*, to *feel* and to *entice*. It is intended as a counter to human exceptionalist modes of thinking, which prioritise abstract, anthropocentric and de-situated ways of knowing.

12 shrc_hrba_leaflet.pdf (scottishhumanrights.com)

References

Abrams, D. (1996). *The Spell of the Sensuous: Perception and Language in a More-Than-Human World*. New York: Vintage Books.

Alzheimer's Society (2019). *Blue Badge Scheme Extended to People with Hidden Disabilities Including People with Dementia*. London: Alzheimer's Society. Available at: https://www.alzheimers.org.uk/news/2019-08-30/blue-badge-scheme-extended-people-hidden-disabilities-including-people-dementia-30 (Accessed: 8 October 2022).

Barad, K. (2007). *Meeting the Universe Halfway: Quantum Physics and the Entanglement of Matter and Meaning*. Durham: Duke University Press.

Bartlett, R. (2000). Dementia as a disability: Can we learn from disability studies and theory? *Journal of Dementia Care*, 8(5), pp. 33–35.

Berg, M., & Seeber, B. K. (2016). *The Slow Professor: Challenging the Culture of Speed in the Academy*. University of Toronto Press.

Braidotti, R. (2013). *The Posthuman*. Cambridge: Polity Press.

Care Quality Commission (2014). *Cracks in the Pathway Summary*. London: Care Quality Commission. Available at: https://www.cqc.org.uk/sites/default/files/20141009_cracks_in_the_pathway_summary_final_1.pdf (Accessed: 8 October 2022).

CTJ (2022). Gardner & Harris -v- Secretary of State for Health and Social Care. Available at: https://www.judiciary.uk/judgments/gardner-harris-v-secretary-of-state-for-health-and-social-care/ (Accessed: 3 November 2022).

D'Souza, R. (2018). *What's Wrong with Rights? Social Movements, Law and Liberal Imaginations*. London: Pluto Press.

Department of Health and Social Care. (2009). *Living Well with Dementia: a national dementia strategy*. London: Department of Health and Social Care. Available at: https://assets.publishing.service.gov.uk/government/uploads/system/uploads/attachment_data/file/168220/dh_094051.pdf (Accessed: 8 October 2022).

Engel, G (1977). The need for a new medical model: A challenge for biomedicine *Science*, New Series, 196(4286), pp. 129–136. Available at: https://www.healtorture.org/sites/healtorture.org/files/The%20Need%20for%20a%20New%20Medical%20Model%20A%20Challenge%20for%20Biomedicine%20by%20George%20L.%20Engel.pdf (Accessed: 8 October 2022).

Fisher, M. (2009). *Capitalist Realism: Is There No Alternative?* London: Zero Books.

Foucault, M. (1996/2002). *The Order of Things. An Archeology of the Human Sciences*. London & New York: Routledge.

Gilbert, S., Sapp, J., & Tauber, A. I. (2012). A symbiotic view of life: We have never been individuals. *Quarterly Review of Biology*, 87(4), pp. 325–341.

Guzmán, P., Tarin-Carrasco, P., Morales-Suarez-Varela, M. and Jiménez-Guerrero, P. (2022). Effects of air pollution over Europe for present and future climate change scenarios. *Environmental Research*, 204(Part A). https://doi.org/10.1016/j.envres.2021.112012 (Accessed: 8 October 2022).

Gwilliam, C., & Gilliard, J (1996). Dementia and the social model of disability. *Journal of Dementia Care*, 4(1), pp. 14–15.

Haraway, D. (2008). *When Species Meet*: Minneapolis: University of Minnesota Press.

Haraway, D. (2016). *Staying with The Trouble: Making Kin in the Chthulucene*. Durham: Duke University Press.

Hendriks, I., Van Vliet, D., Gerritsen, D. and Dröes, R (2016). Nature and dementia: Development of a person-centred approach. *International Psychogeriatrics*, 28(9), pp. 1455–1470. https://doi.org/10.1017/S1041610216000612 (Accessed: 8 October 2022).

Hughes, J. and Williamson, T (2019). *The Dementia Manifesto; Putting Values-based Practice to Work*. Cambridge: Cambridge University Press.

Kirtley, A., & Williamson, T. (2016). *'What is Truth?' An Inquiry about Truth and Lying in Dementia Care*. London: Mental Health Foundation. Available at: https://www.mentalhealth.org.uk/sites/default/files/2022-09/MHF-dementia-truth-inquiry-report.pdf (Accessed: 8 October 2022).

Kitwood, T. (1997). *Dementia Reconsidered: The Person Comes First*. Buckingham: Open University Press.

Latimer, J. (2014). *Joanna Latimer on Wolfe, Barad and Posthuman Ethics*. https://www.theoryculturesociety.org/joanna-latimer-on-wolfe-barad-and-posthuman-ethics/ (Accessed: 11th November 2020).

Magallanes, C. (2018). 'From rights to responsibilities using legal personhood and guardianship for rivers' (Chapter 14) in M. Betsan, L. Te Aho, and M. Humphries-Kil (eds.), *Responsibility. Law and Governance for Living Well with the Earth*. London: Routledge. https://doi.org/10.4324/9780429467622 (Accessed: 8 October 2022).

Mapes, N., Milton, S., Nicholls, V. and Williamson, T. (2016). *Is it nice outside? Consulting people living with dementia and their carers about engaging with the natural environment*. Natural England Commissioned Reports Number 211. Available at: http://publications.naturalengland.org.uk/publication/5910641209507840 (Accessed: 8 October 2022).

Margulis, L. (1970). *Origin of Eukaryotic Cells: Evidence and Research Implications for a Theory of the Origin and Evolution of Microbial, Plant, and Animal Cells on the Precambrian Earth*. New Haven: Yale University Press.

McShane, K (2018). Loving an Unfamiliar World: Dementia, Mental Illness and Climate Change. *Ethics and the Environment*, 23(1), pp. 1–16. https://doi.org/10.2979/ethicsenviro.23.1.01 (Accessed: 8 October 2022).

Mental Health Foundation (2015). *Dementia, rights and the social model of disability*. London: Mental Health Foundation. Available at: https://www.mentalhealth.org.uk/sites/default/files/2022-09/MHF-dementia-rights-policy-discussion.pdf (Accessed: 8 October 2022).

Martino, A. S., & Lindsay, S. M. (2020). Introduction: The intersections of critical disability studies and critical animal studies. *Canadian Journal of Disability Studies*, 9(2), 1–9.

McGettrick, S., & Williamson, T. (2015). *Dementia, Rights and the Social Model of Disability*. London: Mental Health Foundation.

National Audit Office (2007). *Improving services and support for people with dementia*. London: The Stationary Office. Available at: https://www.nao.org.uk/wp-content/uploads/2007/07/0607604es.pdf (Accessed: 8 October 2022).

National Audit Office (2013). *Improving Dementia Services in England – an Interim Report*. London: The Stationary Office. Available at: https://www.nao.org.uk/wp-content/uploads/2010/01/091082es.pdf (Accessed: 8 October 2022).

O'Donnell, E. (2020) Rivers as living beings: Rights in law, but no rights to water? *Griffith Law Review*, 29(4), 643–668. Abstract available at: https://www.tandfonline.com/doi/full/10.1080/10383441.2020.1881304 (Accessed: 8 October 2022)

O'Donnell, E. L., & Talbot-Jones, J (2018). Creating legal rights for rivers: lessons from Australia, New Zealand, and India. *Ecology and Society*, 23(1). Available at: https://www.jstor.org/stable/26799037 (Accessed: 8 October 2022)

Pecharroman, L.C. (2018). Rights of Mature: Rivers that can stand in court. *Resources* 2018, 7(1), 13. https://doi.org/10.3390/resources7010013 (Accessed: 8 October 2022).

Press Association (2018) New blue badge rules to benefit people with hidden disabilities, *The Guardian*, 21 January. Available at: https://www.theguardian.com/society/2018/jan/21/new-blue-badge-parking-permit-rules-benefit-people-autism-dementia-hidden-disabilities (Accessed: 8 October 2022).

Quinn, J., & Blandon, C. (2020). *Lifelong Learning and Dementia: A Posthumanist Perspective*. London: Palgrave Macmillan.

Rahman, S., & Swaffer, K (2018) Assets-based approaches and dementia-friendly communities, *Dementia*, 17(2), pp. 131–137. https://doi.org/10.1177/1471301217751533 (Accessed: 8 October 2022).

Schrader A (2010) Responding to *Pfiesteria piscicida* (the fish killer): Phantomatic ontologies, indeterminacy, and responsibility in toxic microbiology. *Social Studies of Science*, 40(2), pp. 275–306.

Shakespeare, T., Zeilig, H. and Mittler, P. (2019). Rights in mind: Thinking differently and dementia and disability. *Dementia*, 18(3), pp. 1075–1088. Available at: https://researchonline.lshtm.ac.uk/id/eprint/4650612/1/Rights-in-mind.pdf (Accessed: 8 October 2022).

Shannon, K., Bail, K. and Neville, S. (2019). Dementia-friendly community initiatives: An integrative review. *Journal of Clinical Nursing*, 28(11–12), pp. 2035–2045. https://doi.org/10.1111/jocn.14746 (Accessed: 8 October 2022).

Stein, P.J.S. and Stein, M.A. (2022). Disability, human rights and climate justice. *Human Rights Quarterly*, 44(1), pp. 81–110. https://doi.org/10.1353/hrq.2022.0003 (Accessed: 8 October 2022).

Suárez-González, A., Livingston, G., Low, L.F., Cahill, S., Hennelly, N., Dawson, W.D., Weidner, W., Bocchetta, M., Ferri, C.P., Matias-Guiu, J.A., Alladi, S., Musyimi, CW, and Comas-Herrera, A (2020). *Impact and mortality of COVID-19 on people living with dementia: Cross-country report. International Long Term Care Policy Network.* Available at: https://ltccovid.org/wp-content/uploads/2020/08/International-report-on-the-impact-of-COVID-19-on-people-living-with-dementia-19-August-2020.pdf (Accessed: 8 October 2022).

Tsing, A. (2015). *The Mushroom at the End of the World: On the Possibility of Life in Capitalist Ruins.* Princeton: Princeton University Press.

Voluntary Organisations Disabilities Group (2016). *Dementia, Equity and Rights.* London: Voluntary Organisations Disabilities Group. Available at: https://www.vodg.org.uk/wp-content/uploads/2016-VODG-Dementia-equity-and-rights-report.pdf (Accessed: 8 October 2022).

Watts Belser, J. (2020) Disability, Climate Change, and Environmental Violence: The Politics of Invisibility and the Horizon of Hope. *Disability Studies Quarterly*, 40(40). https://doi.org/10.18061/dsq.v40i4.6959 (Accessed: 8 October 2022).

Wei, Y., Wang, Y., Lin, C., Yin, K., Shi, L., Li, L., Zanobetti, A. and Schwartz, J.D. (2019) Associations between seasonal temperature and dementia-associated hospitalizations in New England. *Environmental International*, 126, pp. 228–233. https://doi.org/10.1016/j.envint.2018.12.054 (Accessed: 8 October 2022).

Wilkie, R. (2015). Academic 'dirty work': Mapping scholarly labor in a tainted mixed-species field. *Society & Animals*, 23(3), pp. 211–230.

Wilkinson, R., & Pickett, K (2010). *The Sprit Level: Why Equality is Better for Everyone.* London: Penguin.

Williamson, T. (2015a). Dementia, rights and the social model of disability. *The Journal of Dementia Care*, 23(5), 12–13.

Williamson, T. (2015b). Dementia, public health and public policy–making the connections. *Journal of Public Mental Health*, 14(1), 35–37.

Williamson, T. (2016). *Mapping dementia friendly communities across Europe.* European Foundations' Initiative on Dementia Report. Available at: https://www.efid.info/wp-content/uploads/2016/05/Mapping_DFCS_across_Europe_final_v2.pdf (Accessed: 8 October 2022).

Wolfe, C. (2003). *Animal Rites: American Culture, the Discourse of Species, and Posthumanist Theory.* Chicago: The University of Chicago Press.

Wolfe, C. (2010). *What is Posthumanism?* Minneapolis: University of Minnesota Press.

12 Experts by experience

'I don't want to be shaken,
I want to be a shaker'

*Agnes Houston, Nancy McAdam, James McKillop,
and Martin Robertson*
Facilitated by Paula Brown

Introduction

This chapter is based on a discussion by members of the Scottish Dementia Alumni, a peer-support and campaign group, made up of the chapter authors, who collectively have decades of lived experience of dementia and advocacy. The discussion was recorded and transcribed by the book co-editor, James Fletcher, and the transcript was then edited by the group. The chapter begins by outlining our routes into dementia advocacy and the particular importance of companionship in leading us into campaigning. We recall how difficult it was in the early days, when even dementia-related events would automatically exclude people with dementia. Gradually, we got a foot in the door. We note that it is now more possible for people to be involved in dementia advocacy and in research, but sadly there has been less progress with developing post-diagnostic services. Towards the end of the chapter, we reflect on the difficulties of working with other organisations, which we are keen to do, while also maintaining our independence. We talk about some of our positive experiences, as well as some instances where we have had to move away from collaborations to further our advocacy.

Campaigning and companionship

James: I was diagnosed with multi-infarct dementia last century. At that time, post-diagnosis support was limited to being told: 'You've got up to six years to live, go home and put your affairs in order.' I hid in my house for a while because of fear and shame. After I was diagnosed, Brenda Vincent, who worked in Alzheimer Scotland as a benefits advisor came to see me, to complete forms that I had obtained a year before, read and tossed aside as being irrelevant to me. She explained how to complete the form, and I was awarded some benefit. She had a stall for Alzheimer Scotland at Glasgow City Chambers, which was usually around November each year, selling Christmas goodies. She said I could come and help, as I had stopped going out, and did not converse much with anyone. I wasn't keen, as I could no longer count money in loose change, and I had lost the knack of talking. She didn't mind and said I could

DOI: 10.4324/9781003290353-18

come and stick price labels on goods. She was very persuasive, so I turned up. To my utter astonishment, I found that I was gradually able to talk to potential customers. I became like a barker and enticed the public to stop and admire the goods.

Around then, in early 2000, Heather Wilkinson wanted to contact people who were newly diagnosed with dementia for research purposes. We met up, and we did the research project. I started to go out to look for company and other people like me. There was nowhere. There was a Scottish Mental Health Foundation, so I went to some of their meetings, and they ostracised me. They told me that I didn't belong there because I didn't have a mental health condition. I argued that I did, I had brain damage, but they didn't want me and I was pushed out. I thought: 'Where do I go? What happens now?' I don't think that the Scottish Mental Health Foundation has changed, because now people with dementia have somewhere else to go.

Somehow the three of us met up, maybe Brenda was escorting me to meet Heather, and we got talking and planning. We mulled over the situation and thought it would be a good idea to start up a group, exclusively for people with dementia. Somewhere we would be safe, and free to voice our thoughts, without fear of being ridiculed. We travelled around Scotland seeking people to join, and there was much excitement, as this was unheard of, people with dementia having a voice of their own. We went about setting up the Scottish Dementia Working Group (SDWG). That was for people with dementia only. The Glasgow Dementia Group was actually started first, but it closed after a year because there were no funds. We built up the SDWG as a place where you can have your say without fear of someone jumping on you.

Nancy: I joined about two years after James, in 2004. I can remember going to meetings and they were in huge halls with space for six or seven different areas. We collected food from people because we had lunch before we had meetings. We ended up with four or five tables of people. Some of the Highland group even came to visit us one of the times. I was actually a campaigner already. I got arrested for campaigning about GM crops and protesting at the town hall, so I had form. You go to a lot of effort to do it, to get arrested and go through all that trauma in some way. Campaigning with the Alumni is very different. We're on Zoom. That's what I struggle with now, when I try to get myself on Microsoft Teams. Campaigning now involves an awful lot of technology that I'm not good with.

Agnes: I came along about seven years after James, in 2007. He was chairing the SDWG. By that time, nothing had really changed from James' experience because I was treated exactly the same way when I was diagnosed. I know that the SDWG had been working hard and doing things, but at the local level there was nothing. There were no dementia cafés, there was nothing. You were told to go home, and you just sat in a corner. Nobody assisted you with anything. You only got a nurse if you were on Aricept or a cognitive enhancer. I personally believed that Alzheimer Scotland was the be all and end all of everything. I didn't know any different. I didn't know there was anything else other than Alzheimer Scotland. It was the only name I'd heard.

One day an Alzheimer Scotland care worker came to my dad's home, because my dad also had dementia, and he asked me how I was. I burst into tears because nobody had ever asked me how I was since I'd been diagnosed. Everybody was always talking to me and about me. He told me about the SDWG and suggested that I needed to meet others who I would fit in with. He took me along, and when I came in, they were all sitting round a table with James chairing it. I thought that he had taken me to the wrong room because I couldn't tell who had dementia. They were all talking and laughing. They were advocating and they were passionate. I couldn't believe that it was real.

Then for a couple of years I followed James around like a puppy, trying to get a bit of what he had. I wanted Nancy's laughter and zest for life too. It was really a wonderful experience. Although it was a campaigning group, it was also the only thing available for me. I had to become a campaigner to be part of the SDWG, and I've never looked back. It's like Kitwood said – love is at the heart of it. I always say that the SDWG loved me better, because when I went along, I was loved by the people with dementia. I was accepted by them as I was. James and the others joke that the worst thing they ever did was to teach me and enable me to find my voice again and to speak. I had word-finding problems and you wouldn't recognise me as the same person that I am today. They laughed at me when I wanted to ask someone to pass the sugar and I couldn't get the words out, so I'd click my fingers. They laughed because it was all okay and they didn't care. They allowed me to express myself and they told me that I didn't need to try to use big words anymore. Although we're talking about campaigning and advocacy, there was peer support there, just not in those words. I don't think I ever heard the words 'peer support' mentioned. We just helped one another, and we just did what we had to do. My first job in the SDWG was as a meet and greeter. I was giving people wee badges and directing people. The people from Aberdeen sat on one table, the people from Dundee on another, Glasgow on another and so on.

James: One of the outstanding things that I remember about the SDWG meetings was how big they were. About 60 people would come to our meetings in Dundee. Agnes would greet every single one with a hug and a smile. She was the best ambassador that I've known, then and since.

Martin: I started off as a campaigner. I chained myself to bulldozers on a bypass. I couldn't get arrested because I was a board member of Friends of the Earth, and we had lots of lawyers. Others could get arrested but I had to be careful where I went and what I did. That's where I got my campaigning spirit from. I was first diagnosed with dementia down in

England, and there was nothing down there at all. We moved up to Scotland in 2017. Even then, in 2017, the GP and the older person's consultant didn't signpost me anywhere. Luckily, I'm tech savvy, so I just looked things up, but especially in rural areas, people won't come to you. You have to go out and find them.

A foot in the door

Agnes: Martin and Nancy were campaigners, but I wasn't a campaigner until dementia. It was frustration and anger that led to me becoming a campaigner, especially how members had to give so much of their time. Nancy was travelling down from the Black Isle to Edinburgh to work with the government when they were doing their first National Dementia Strategy, and they put her up in a noisy hostel. We put ourselves out when there weren't many of us that were willing to campaign at that level, and at the boring meetings. We were uncomfortable. We weren't well looked after. There was no meet and greet at the train. You had to make your own way there and find your own way back. I remember one time getting lost and nobody could find me, and it was late at night before I could get home. The people who are getting diagnosed now don't know how good it is to campaign now. When James started campaigning, and then Nancy and I were going out campaigning, it was hard. It was really tough, and we were not welcomed with open arms.

James: I've actually written a piece on valuing people with dementia (see McKillop 2021) that tells similar tales to what happened to Agnes and Nancy when they were initially campaigning. There are some really horrifying tales of what happened and how we were treated. For example, in 2000 I heard there was an Alzheimer's conference in Glasgow. I tried to go and they wouldn't let me in because I had dementia. I had a support worker called Brenda and she managed to get me a photographer badge, so I got in as a photographer. People disregarded you. They treated you like you were dirt.

Agnes: I didn't know anything about campaigning. I would push myself into meetings because I wanted to hear what they were saying. Some days in the SDWG we would go to four meetings in one day, all over Scotland. We were jumping on trains and coming home at night, sometimes with no lunch.

James: One day I did a talk to social workers in Perth. I left Glasgow, went to Perth by bus, did my talk, got the bus to Edinburgh, joined some sort of meeting, got a train to Motherwell, joined a board meeting there, then home late at night. I've had worse than that. Dr Alzheimer diagnosed the illness that bears his name in 1906 (see Fletcher's discussion of the historic development of Alzheimer's disease in Chapter 1). I personally think that after 100 years of Alzheimer's we've got to do things for ourselves, not to have people keep doing everything for us. I wonder if I hadn't come along if that would still be the case. We had to come and do these things because nobody was doing it, not Alzheimer Scotland nor anybody.

Agnes: I think what happened was we learnt. It was like being an apprentice. We were learning on the job. We were seeing how people were behaving and how we should behave. If we were asked to talk anywhere or we were representing the group, we prepared ourselves extremely well. We read up and it took a lot of work to prepare our heads for what we were doing. We were going into these things on our own the majority of the time, and we were sitting in there and breaking down barriers. We were gaining respect over the years.

Martin: I see it as you having broken down the door, and now we're in the room because of you. That is how I look at it. Without those early struggles people like me would not be in the room today, so it is up to us to carry it on. Due to the Alumni and the Life Changes Trust, I am gobsmacked by just how many things I am actually involved with. That is partly down to the Alumni, and then the other things I have just pushed my way onto.

Debating progress

James: I don't know how much things have improved. These days I don't have much contact with people who have been newly diagnosed, and I think since the Covid-19 lockdowns fewer people have been diagnosed, so it is difficult for me to say. I do know that we fought for post-diagnostic support. I'm not saying that access to it is good, because it's not good, but at least we fought for it and we won a guarantee from the government.

Martin: The guarantee is absolutely totally useless. We have a 20% post-diagnostic support rate up here in Aberdeenshire. What we really need is a step change where the consultant gives out a diagnosis, they also give out some knowledge. It can even be just signposting forward to organisations, giving people the opportunity to reach out. Then if they want to do it, they can do it. That is what we should be aiming for. I don't think that I would have been able to do this in the 2000s, but I go along to all the local authority meetings. I'm a member of a dedicated subgroup. Earlier campaigning has opened that door and now I'm using it. Some things are better. Our access is better now, but on the ground it's very much still a postcode lottery I'm afraid. It is a bugbear of mine, but much of the central belt of Scotland is a lot better off than remoter areas.

Agnes: This is where I would agree that it is a postcode lottery. I feel that access has certainly got better. There are more groups because of the turnaround in government attitudes. If you're setting something up around dementia and you want some funding it is now expected that you should have a person living with dementia on your committee, whereas we had to push our way in. We had to do it nicely and politely at first and then to start putting across our point of view in a more assertive way. Has it changed? If you'd have asked me three weeks ago, I'd have said yes. There is post-diagnostic support. There are dementia cafés and meeting centres here and there, but it definitely remains a postcode lottery. I was asked to a yoga wellness hub, to speak to people living with dementia, their carers and professionals, etc. I thought everybody knew about the basics, such as being able to apply to get your council tax paid for. Nobody knew about it. None of them knew about the cards that James has introduced, that say: 'I have dementia. Here are my issues. Etc.' Nobody had even heard about the Iris Murdoch Centre at Stirling University. I thought... I could have cried, and I came home feeling very despondent. I wondered what we had been doing for fifteen years. With all this running around and campaigning, what is happening?

James: Just to be clear, the University of Stirling and the Iris Murdoch centre are two separate entities. They are joined by a corridor, but they are two separate entities. I was quite involved with the Iris Murdoch centre. I went and gave presentations to people who came for training. I think I was doing training for social work students at the University of Stirling for a few years, but I can no longer do presentations.

Nancy: I gave my first talk at Stirling, with Phillip Bryers supporting me through it all, and June Andrews was the person who introduced me as a person with dementia.

Martin: They now use videos of us, so we are there for posterity.

Agnes: There is still a lot of work that needs to be done. We need to stop talking to the people who already get it. We need to get out there and speak to the people who don't know about it. That's where the campaigning needs to go, to the areas that have got nothing, like North Lanarkshire where I come from. I'm sure there are hundreds of other areas like it. Martin has been a great asset to us in terms of showing us what it's like to be diagnosed now and the changing faces of dementia.

Martin: There's a lot of tokenism going on. People will take one of us on board just to say that they've got somebody living with dementia on board. That happens a lot. Also, funding tends to go to places that already exist because it's easier to show a flagship. Nothing gets nothing, but something gets something. That's my view. For instance, there are two main organisations in Scotland but I don't feel that either of them truly represent my views accurately, so I'm finding it hard as an independent voice. The Scottish Dementia Alumni amplifies my voice and the group's unique voice.

Agnes: It goes back to the question of has anything changed. There's a lot of work still to be done. Things have changed in some ways, but in other ways very little has changed. Are people with dementia still forcing themselves on to committees? Yes, they are. They're just no longer having to pretend to be photographers to get inside. One big change has been getting some financial recognition for our work, through the ECREDibles group. The ECREDibles is a peer-support group for people who are interested in research. It is made up of nine people with dementia that sit alongside Edinburgh academics, and we can do as much or as little within the research field as we want, and we are actually tackling our own research questions. That is something that has changed. Even if we can't take money because of our benefits, we can get vouchers. I got supermarket vouchers recently. In fact, I've had them twice. I do Chinese cooking online and I've bought a wok with the vouchers. Every time I use it, I'm reminded of the work that I do, and everything tastes better because of it.

Martin: That is something that the Life Changes Trust helped to get going. They have taught us how to co-research and how to get the skills. The Life Changes Trust has financed all of that. I think that that started a ball rolling with co-researching. Dr Rosalie Ashworth is really into it, working with Partners in Research. We wrote a book together and co-researching emerged out of that, using it in the academic world and getting it out there (Ashworth et al. in press; see also Ashworth & Partners in Research 2022).

Agnes: There is the Dementia Enquirers project as well, developing co-research and research led by people living with dementia. They have the pioneers group that I'm part of. The pioneers have allies, Rosalie Ashworth, Tom Shakespeare, etc. who sat around the table and helped us to get funding to give to other groups. The pioneers are all people living with dementia, along with allies who keep us right with the academia side. We put a call out through the Dementia Enquirers project for applications, which we received from other groups, detailing what they wanted to do. I remember the Alumni put one in and we had to jump through hoops to get it, because we wrote guidelines and gold standards. It all came from people living with dementia working with renowned academics who facilitated it and enabled us to do it. That was the first time that I realised that the book about Self-Management that we were writing with the Life Changes Trust, as a research project, we couldn't have got it officially recognised as research because we weren't backed by a university. We still followed research guidance and did our own research, nonetheless.

Maintaining independence

Agnes: The SDWG had vibrant and wonderful meetings. It was totally independent. That is a very important word because at the moment there are not too many truly independent voices of people with dementia, and truly independent groups. When James was chairing the SDWG, right up until 2013, we were independent.

Eventually, there came a time when we were long in the tooth. There were new members coming in who had their own issues, and we still weren't getting our issues addressed. When we made suggestions to the people who were supposedly facilitating our voices to be heard, they then had to go back to their employers to have it approved. It was a strange thing. I'll never forget being at the meeting where they were talking about changing the constitution that James and SDWG founders had written. The organisation thought that we should adopt their constitution and that we didn't need a constitution of our own. The new members didn't get it because they didn't get the history. I could see the people that I knew who had died during the campaigning, and I could hear their voices saying that we were selling them down the Swanee. We shouldn't let this happen. We needed a backbone. We needed to stand up and fight it. When you're in a democratic group and it's put to a vote, no matter how passionate you are about it, you have to go with the flow.

It was then that I thought that something important had changed. We were not independent anymore. We were being told and we were puppets. That's what the Alumni evolved out of. I spoke to James and asked him if he would come along with me if I found a new place. At that time, we didn't have anything. We had no funding. We'd nowhere to hang our hats. He said yes because we could still be part of the SDWG. We've got nothing against them. We just had to think about what happened to us and where we were to go to deal with our issues and the things that we were facing as our dementias were progressing.

James: That was when we were saying: What about the people who had been diagnosed for years? What about the people who were completely abandoned?

Agnes: That was when we couch surfed. We started in a café and we had no budget. My daughter came along, and she facilitated it. She took minutes to keep track of where we were going. We had to spend the first year licking our wounds because a lot of us had been traumatised by what was happening. We had given years to the campaign, and there was still a lot of campaigning left in us, but we didn't know how we could do it, kindly, in parallel with other groups. That was the start of the Alumni. The name came from someone in England at one of the big events. I mentioned needing a name for our group and someone suggested 'the Alumni.' I took it back to the group and they thought it was great, so that's how we adopted 'the Alumni.' Then it was a year later before we found a place to hang our hat. First of all, it was a place called ALISS. We had two meetings there and they gave us a room, but they couldn't guarantee it, so we never had a day. That went on for two or three months in the winter.

Then I was in Europe, and European people thought that Scotland is brilliant, and I told them that all the well-known faces from Scotland didn't have anywhere to hang our hats. That was when Irene Oldfather came up to me. She looked embarrassed, and she said that the Alliance Trust would give us a room. We never looked back after that. Two years later my daughter took ill, and there was one of the previous group members called Rosemary, who we all knew, who had been widowed. I phoned her up and asked her if she would come to help us, just to jot down what we were doing and make tea and sandwiches. That's how it all started. It was a wing and a prayer, and we've never looked back. We just didn't want to lose our independence. That was the big, big thing about it all – people could support us but not speak for us. That was the philosophy. It took us a year to lick our wounds and talk about it. Then we were asked to join the Dementia Engagement and Empowerment Project (DEEP) (members of which have co-authored Chapter 3). They came and spoke to us and we really put them through the wringer. That was when we decided that this was a good way to go forward and so we became part of the DEEP network.

Martin: The Life Changes Trust has kept us going. We've done the hard work but they've allowed us to have our own Facilitator, who does everything behind the scenes, a personal assistant named Paula. The good thing is that she is ours. She's not paid by an outsider. That is so vital, that she's independent and not a professional from a local authority or a health worker. There is so much difference that comes with that and it is an important point to get across. We're kind of employers. That is important because she doesn't have her own agenda and doesn't speak for us. With her help and the support of the Life Changes Trust we've published a book about GPs (Scottish Dementia Alumni 2021a). We took a booklet called 'Knowledge is Power' (Caban Bangor University Educators et al. 2020) that was originally from Wales and reworked it to apply to Scotland (The Beacon Club et al. 2021), because there are a lot of differences in Scotland when it comes to health services. We've also written a booklet called 'Dementia and Preparing for the Unexpected' (Scottish Dementia Alumni 2021b). We've just started writing a booklet on sleep challenges, funded by the University of Exeter (Scottish Dementia Alumni forthcoming), as well as a game to try to engage children (collaborating with the excellent Science Ceilidh) so that we can work more intergenerationally.

Agnes: Life Changes Trust made a big difference in Scotland by giving small grants to independent groups. The big charities were the only game in town, and you had to assimilate to be a part of them, to act in specific ways. If your views didn't align with the organisation, you weren't invited in. Life Changes Trust gave the Alumni the freedom to be ourselves and to create our own group in our own time. They did that through a collection of peer-to-peer support grants. They also helped us to put the applications for the funding in because we'd never done anything like that before. From there we just did what we do best. We started to write these booklets, starting with the one on self-management.

I went to Life Changes Trust and told them that the legacy of our campaigning was being lost and asked if we could get a history written about it. We had previously tried it but I don't think that it was a true reflection. It was a great start, but it wasn't quite right. With funding from the Life Changes Trust, Philly Hare from Innovations in Dementia wrote 'Loud and Clear', which is all about the rise of dementia campaigning (Hare 2020). It wasn't just about the SDWG. It covers a whole host of different things and it's a brilliant book. It provided a timeline and I'm keen to do something similar for the Alumni.

Negotiating organisations

Martin: I can see problems ahead. I feel that it's very important to maintain our independence and not to be swallowed up by larger groups.

Agnes: Only if the people living with dementia allow it. Facilitators need to leave any organisational agendas at the door. As a person living with dementia, you don't really have an understanding of what's going on, and you have to trust these people. People living with dementia have to be empowered to speak up. We need people to support us, keep us right, keep us on time and all those things that are part of facilitating, but facilitators must not take over. Even if they are working for a large organisation, as long as we can get through our agenda then we're not being taken over.

Martin: I wonder about funders too, if we accept funding, we need to make it clear that we are still uniquely independent voices, even if the funder requires us to campaign with them. It will still be with our unique voice.

Agnes: As the Alumni, we need to be a part of the networks to raise our voice in an appropriate way. Sometimes we will say that we are sorry but that this isn't independence, when we can hear the philosophy and sense the influence of an organisation, or if we can see that a certain ethos is taking over. You need to be in it to change it, so you can't take yourself out of it because you're frightened of losing your independence. They can't take our independence away, only if we hand it over to them, and as long as we've got any breath left in our body, we're not going to let that happen. We need to be involved, otherwise how will those new groups know what's going on without our wisdom and past experience? We can't force feed them this wisdom. We can only drip it in every so often, until they have the lightbulb moment. Not everyone in the large organisations are going to understand that, but some of them will. If we are an independent group, then we are free to do what we like. We still need to be involved to make a change, but we don't always need to join them.

We also can't force people to be independent if they don't want to be independent. That's the new dementia now, you've got to be dependent on others. People with dementia today can be at risk of being over-consulted or manipulated by powerful groups. That's why we as the Alumni set out to mentor new groups and speak to people who are newly diagnosed. That was part of our original vision, so that people would gain the wisdom that we've learned over the years. Then they can make their own choices regarding what they want to do, but making those choices with knowledge, because knowledge is power. That's why we are still in the game, and we are still doing this, because we are still having that battle with those that are more powerful and have got big money. That kills me, because when I did my first booklet (Houston 2015), I think it was about £6500 that I got. My daughter took time off and bought a second-hand film camera, having never used one before. We just went out and we were fuelled by passion. We were fuelled by the need. This is necessary. That booklet went international and has been translated into many languages. The funders said it was the best value to investment that they'd ever had. It just went off because the need was there.

Martin: I can give you a few examples of power. There is currently a big splash in the newspapers about dementia getting £1million to go to meeting centres. Of that, less than £250,000 is going to meeting centres directly. I put in a freedom of information request to the government to demand to know what was going on. More of that money is going to learning organisations than is going to meeting centres. Then there is money for an audit. £75,000 goes to admin. There is a total power imbalance here. Less than a quarter of the money is going directly to meeting centres.

Agnes: I think that part of the problem is that we are still a bit naïve. When we are putting our funding bids in, we don't pay ourselves. We do it for free. We need to learn to be paying ourselves, because it would appear that the bigger the bid, the more 'wow factor' the bid has and the more chance that we're going to get it. We should be making bigger funding bids to the Big Lottery and things like that. We could ask for £250,000 and see how we get on. It's not about the money. It's about being recognised for our time and what we bring to the meetings that we're doing.

In Scotland, Alzheimer Scotland can only hand out their own publications. They will not signpost you to anything that they haven't set up. It's dementia advisors that are staffing a lot of these post-diagnostic centres and they're mostly Alzheimer Scotland staff. Those staff are being disempowered because, although they know that our booklets are out there, their managers won't allow them to hand them out. A lot of dementia advisors are handing out the booklets under the table. I really do feel that this has to be addressed. All information, whether or not it is stamped by Alzheimer Scotland, has to be on show. The Welsh version of 'Knowledge is Power' has been available in Wales for a long time, but our Scottish version took ages to come to Scotland and it still isn't officially recognised by Alzheimer Scotland. It isn't rubberstamped by them.

I believe that Scotland was put on the back foot, and we lost a lot of what we had gained. England and Wales have overtaken Scotland now. That's my own personal opinion. Bradford University and Sheffield

University are recognising people living with dementia and giving them doctorates. I backed Edinburgh Centre for Research on the Experience of Dementia. I turned up for years and years and years, and we are now making progress through the ECREDibles research group, a sister group to ECRED that we set up to run in partnership. In my opinion, Scotland has never fully appreciated the amount of work that people have put in to lift them up.

Martin: I think it is changing. At least, the bits that I'm in are changing because I'm changing them. I'm involved now in several funding bids. I've actually been writing funding bids with people for ECRED. Gillian Mathews was already doing something on counselling, and she came to me to help with the funding bid. I'm pushing myself into these things.

Agnes: I'm too tired to push myself into these things now. The counselling project, I sat at that table before it was a fact. I had asked to get counselling, and I was told by my GP that people living with dementia don't get counselling. I raised this at ECRED and made a song and dance. I was at that table, but I was never involved. I was never invited in by Edinburgh University. I believe ECRED made use of my skills. I wanted to sit round that table, so I was aware that it was going on, and I accepted that it was going on so that I could have the information on what was happening in Edinburgh University. I'm not angry about it, but I don't think they should be allowed to do it with others.

Martin: In a way, that encapsulates the difference between us and other groups. I think, with the Alumni, we all share the same values, but I couldn't talk for other groups. I couldn't do it. My voice would show that I wasn't believing what I said. I wouldn't be passionate. I don't like naming other groups but a lot of them are quite happy with where they are in the totem pole. I wouldn't be. I want to be independent and to actually alter the things that matter to me. Other groups will do what they're told. I want to be a mover and a shaker. I don't want to be shaken. I want to shake.

Nancy: Can you rattle and roll too?

References

Ashworth, R. & Partners in Research. (2022). *Partners in Research: An Equal Partnership Approach to 'Patient and Public Involvement'*. Neuroprogressive and Dementia Network: NHS Tayside.

Ashworth, R., Cheung, M., Fyvel, S., Gilder, W., Hay, S., Henry, W., Hill, A., Houston, A., Lamont, M., Maddocks, C., Qureshi, M., Robertson, M. & Ross, D. (in press). *Challenging Assumptions around Dementia: User-led Research and Untold Stories*. UK: Palgrave Publishers.

Caban Bangor University Educators, DEEP United Dwyfor & Meirionnydd & Fuse & Muse Swansea. (2020). *Knowledge Is Power*. https://www.dementiavoices.org.uk/wp-content/uploads/2020/08/Knowledge-is-Power-dementia-booklet.pdf

Hare, P. (2020). *Loud and Clear: Exploring Two Decades of Involvement, Voice and Activism by People with Dementia in Scotland*. https://www.lifechangestrust.org.uk/project/loud-clear-exploring-two-decades-involvement-voice-and-activism-people-dementia-scotland#:~:text=Loud%20and%20Clear'%20tells%20the,Scotland%20confronted%20the%20status%20quo.

Houston, A. (2015). *Dementia & Sensory Challenges*. https://www.lifechangestrust.org.uk/sites/default/files/Leaflet.pdf

McKillop, J. (2021). Valuing people with dementia. *Alzheimer Europe*. https://www.alzheimer-europe.org/news/living-dementia-blog-post-james-mckillop-valuing-people-dementia

Scottish Dementia Alumni. (2021a). *Dementia & GP Services*. https://www.lifechangestrust.org.uk/sites/default/files/publication/files/GP%20Project%20%20Digital%20Final.pdf

Scottish Dementia Alumni. (2021b). *Dementia & Preparing for the Unexpected*. https://www.dementiavoices.org.uk/wp-content/uploads/2016/10/Preparing-for-the-Unexpected-FINAL-digital-.pdf

Scottish Dementia Alumni. (forthcoming). *Dementia and Sleep Challenges*.

The Beacon Club., Dementia Voices East Dunbartonshire., Scottish Dementia Alumni. & STAND in Fife. (2021). *Knowledge is Power Scotland*. https://www.dementiavoices.org.uk/wp-content/uploads/2021/04/Knowledge_is_Power_English_booklet_single_A5_pages_AW.pdf

Conclusion

Multi-Disciplinary, multi-historied, multi-critical

James Rupert Fletcher and Andrea Capstick

(Un)disciplining histories

We introduced this collection by cautioning against simplistic approaches to history, imposing artificially linear narratives of progress and/or decline onto histories that are better interpreted as multiple and fluid, and can often appear somewhat contradictory. As Andrea Capstick notes in her chapter, dementia studies have often been found wanting when it comes to nurturing sophisticated historical sensibilities. It has been our intention to challenge that deficiency. Hopefully, in light of the preceding chapters, the reader will now have a stronger sense of historical multiplicity. In this concluding chapter, we find it helpful to apply a similar analysis to dementia studies itself, particularly in reference to the nature of what is 'critical' and what is not. The seemingly separate aims of defining (critical) dementia studies and defining its history (and doing both together from a critical perspective) are inextricably bound up with one another. Indeed, the criticality of this history is largely predicated on an alertness to and embracing of a distinct lack of definitiveness; a sense in which the past is far from finished and static, but is instead something that we should make and remake as a dementia studies community, just as we do dementia studies itself.

The self-storying of dementia studies often relates an origin story whereby the late 1980s and early 1990s was a key time, during which psychosocially minded scholars developed anti-(bio)medical critiques (see James Fletcher's chapter 1). That work remains highly influential today, but the reiteration of such histories as though they are moments of ex-nihilo insight and resistance obscures a messier past. To begin with, there are questions about when we stop chasing the lengthening shadows cast by all social theory. For instance, one might reasonably argue that any robust history must trace Tom Kitwood's ideas back to Carl Roger's (1946) client-centred psychology and Martin Buber's (1923 [1937]) philosophy of dialogue, the medicalisation thesis back to deviance sociologists (Conrad 1975), the ordering of intersubjectivities back to George Mead's (1934) interactionist philosophy. Likewise, parallel developments can be traced through the same timepoints. For example, Nancy Harding and Colin Palfrey (1997) published a text on the social construction of dementia the same year that Tom Kitwood (1997) published Dementia Reconsidered, the former offering a sociological interpretation that both

DOI: 10.4324/9781003290353-19

converged and diverged with the latter. In each instance, the historian of a particular disciplinary persuasion must draw artificial lines in both time and thought to prevent an increasingly fruitless meandering ever backwards and ever outwards. Contemporary engagement with dementia across the social sciences and humanities sits amidst an infinite web of influences, and one could feasibly trace countless paths across its face.

This is true of what we might consider the historical influences on something that would become dementia studies, but it is also true of scholarship attending to dementia more explicitly. It is certainly misleading to view the past several decades as unique in this respect. For instance, a rich tradition of American social psychology spoke to dementia in the mid-20th century, situating it within sociopolitical circumstances and contributing to associated legal transformations (Ballenger 2017). Before that, psychiatrists in the early 20th century developed robust critiques of emerging disease-based formulations of Alzheimer's disease, which they deemed problematic by virtue of being stripped from the wider context of ageing (Fuller 1912). This developed into 1930s psychological accounts predicated on a lack of convincing biogenic aetiology (Rothschild & Trainor 1937). Travelling further back still to the early 19th century, Phillippe Pinel (1806) characterised senile dementia in primarily emotional terms rather than as being attributed to disease per se. Retrospectively, this imagining of cognitive impairment in later life feels poignant to dementia studies more than 200 years later. Hence, the contemporary historian can pursue a certain resemblance of dementia studies far into the past, and the results of such pursuit are indebted to the disposition of the pursuer.

From this description, it should begin to become evident that the difficulty of laying out a conventional mechanistic history (i.e. A begot B begot C) is twofold. Firstly, history is not really like this. It is multiple, messy and perpetually vulnerable to re-imagination. Secondly, and similarly, dementia studies is itself nowhere near as definitive as one might assume given its contemporary institutionalisation in journals, edited collections, associations, university programmes, etc. As this volume exemplifies, scholars from a wide range of disciplinary backgrounds apply many different approaches and methods to an eclectic array of dementia-related issues. The psychologist interviewing care workers, the literary scholar analysing a graphic novel, the activist speaking about their sensory disorder – these are all the happenings of a heterogeneous dementia studies that is perpetually shapeshifting. All our explanation is therefore temporary and contingent. In a manner of bricolage, we explain phenomena by using the concepts and 'knowledges' that are currently available to us; the tools we have to hand (Lévi-Strauss 1962 [1966]). One inspiring implication of this recognition is that there are almost certainly many more affinities that are yet to be remarked upon, between scholars in different traditions working on different topics, but nonetheless travelling similar journeys; that is, troubling dementia as a sociopolitical entity. In this book, we have attempted to give at least a taste of the panoply of traditions, standpoints and conceptualisations that flow through and enliven dementia studies as a space where anthropologists, activists and artists come together.

This book is in some sense a history of critical dementia studies and a history of oscillating critical sensibilities within dementia studies, but it is also intended to be a critical approach to cultivating a history, or histories, of dementia studies. To this end, it is not sufficient to merely trouble the nature of disciplinary history, dementia studies and entanglements of the two. More than this, a critical historical approach should recognise that our ongoing efforts to divine, play around with and rearticulate disciplinary and temporal boundaries are themselves forms of political action. For example, the commonplace regurgitation of linear histories – flowing neatly from Alois Alzheimer's 1900s work, through 1960s electron-microscopy, 1990s amyloid hypotheses and 2010s drug development (Herrup 2021) – effectively solidifies an artificially spotless narrative of progress. This has practical implications. It obscures the many pockets of resistance and counter-narratives that shared each of those timepoints (Fletcher 2021a). In opposition to this obscuration, the act of making histories multiple and messy, coupled with a resistance to prioritising particular histories (especially progress narratives), can furnish some of the intellectual foundations necessary for pursuing critical dementia studies today. For instance, the traditional veneration of Alois Alzheimer's seminal work can be tempered by acknowledging the silencing of his contemporary critics, particularly in reference to institutional racism (Powell 2019). Similarly, the recent successes of public awareness raising are repeatedly lauded, yet we might trouble this progress narrative by asking why, as awareness has apparently increased, dementia has simultaneously become one of the public's most feared conditions (Fletcher 2021b). This idea of resistively manipulating multiple histories as a critical and generative practice is returned to below, but first some reflection on another core qualification – 'critical' – is necessary.

'Critical' affinities and frictions

If the question of 'dementia studies' as a meaningful historical entity is challenging, then tying down something akin to a '*critical* dementia studies' is an almost Sisyphean task. While compiling this text in collaboration with numerous dementia scholars, it has been consistently apparent to us as editors that there are a variety of views across the field regarding what qualifies any given iteration of dementia studies as being properly critical. This is not helped by the ubiquity of appeals to being 'critical' across much contemporary social scientific and humanities scholarship in general. As a route into unpacking this issue, we can break down the various points of view that we have encountered into three very crude flavours of critical-adjacency, each of which is represented in this book. That said, it is vital to acknowledge that in reality the particularities of what one does and does not consider critical vary far more considerably, to the extent that there is certainly no definitive answer. It seems unlikely that any consensus will be reached in this respect, but as we will conclude, this is not necessarily a problem.

For some commentators, simply critiquing the (bio)medical model and advocating something more in line with a social model, or even a biopsychosocial model, is sufficient to render scholarship critical. From this perspective, the majority of work discussed herein, if not all of it, appears to be distinctly critical. Early work on personhood and selfhood certainly makes the cut by virtue of its relocating dementia in the social world and decentring steadfast biogenic determinism. There is some logic to the conviction that critiques of (bio)medicalisation are inherently critical. For those of us who have come of age as dementia scholars in an intellectual context already replete with critiques of 1990s psychosocial work, it is perhaps easy to dismiss how radical such projects have been. There are scholars still in the field who can recall a pre-Kitwood world, and therefore perhaps have a stronger sense of how impactful those theoretical developments were at the time. Moreover, for lecturers who introduce social scientific work on (bio)medicalisation and personhood to health professionals for the first time, the criticality and radicalness of the core ideas remains palpably vibrant today. In their chapter, Jackie Kindell, Aagje Swinnen and John Keady are clear that it is vital not to prematurely dispose of such commitments in a rush towards enticing new forms of the critical.

From a second standpoint, it is an attentiveness to the sociopolitical, however conceived, that renders some dementia studies scholarship authentically critical. It is here that we begin to see an explicit pulling apart of critical and a non-critical dementia studies. From this perspective, a focus on intersubjectivities irrespective of political contexts is at best naïve, and at worst actively perpetuates some of the harmful facets of dementia that associated scholarship should seek to resist (Bartlett & O'Connor 2010). This argument, which is developed across citizenship and human rights literatures, relies on a social scientific use of 'critical theory' in the orthodox sense. Hence, a critical approach demarcates an indebtedness to the critical theory tradition of the Frankfurt school, emphasising a commitment to challenging norms and transformative politics (Horkheimer 1972; How 2017). Besides traditional scholarship, the endeavours of dementia activists, such as those described in the Alumni's chapter, can also readily be situated in this area of dementia studies.

Finally, there are those who argue that any dementia scholarship that remains grounded in and even devoted to humanism cannot be truly critical because it perpetuates a set of normative political commitments that disadvantage people with dementia, even as well-intentioned self-identifying critical scholars seek to use that humanism as a form of emancipation (see Toby Williamson and Nick Jenkins' chapter for a debate between proponents of the second and third position). As with the other two standpoints, there is certainly something to this posthumanist perspective. In his advocacy of its merits, Jenkins offers evidence that posthumanism can be used to challenge fundamental norms that determine dementia and to agitate for associated political transformations. In Toby Williamson's responses to these arguments, we gain an appreciation of what is at stake, and perhaps learn something of the rabbit hole down which such debates have the potential to lead us. Is it critical to apply a critical approach to a critical approach? Or is this anti-critical? Or perhaps both at once? There are also important questions to be asked of approaches rooted in posthumanism and new materialism regarding the extent to which they are able to be practically critical. By downplaying human agency, such approaches seemingly shut down possibilities for politically deliberative transformative action in the manner advocated by traditional critical theory.

One of the key causes for uncertainty here is that the contexts to which the dual commitments of critical theory correspond are constantly shifting. Criticality is somewhat ephemeral because it speaks to temporally bound political contexts, after all, it was once critical to agitate against the killing of witches. If a critical scholar successfully challenges norms and implements political transformation, does this mean that the critical project is complete, or does that action simply lay the ground for future critical work? For example, if we were to successfully develop a response to dementia grounded in and fully respecting citizenship, would our critical project be fulfilled, or would a new critical scholarship be required to drive a new phase of transformation targeting the new citizenship-based reality? This uncertainty resonates throughout this volume and the previous volume in this series (Ward & Sandberg 2023), speaking directly to the nature of what it is that dementia studies seeks to achieve. As we have stated and will restate, it seems fair to characterise this basic aim as being to unsettle dementia as a contingent political entity.

These tensions matter in a very practical sense. Barbara Prainsack (2014: 652) notes that '[t]he key to ... medicine that fosters solidarity and is sensitive to people's needs lies in being cautious about what idea of personhood we use and promote'. The manner in which we frame the nature of people affected by dementia inevitably has profound implications for how those people are treated, an observation that is exemplified throughout this collection. Jackie Kindell, Aagje Swinnen and John Keady caution against hastily discarding personhood-focused therapeutic approaches, because these represent a profound improvement on some of the earlier practices that Keady himself recalls. Considering more politically minded scholarships, Moïse Roche, Maria Zubair and James Fletcher regret the tendency for well-intentioned engagements with race and ethnicity to inadvertently exacerbate minoritisation and its harmful effects, often by failing to attend to the types of status that are being ascribed to research subjects. Turning to human rights scholarship, in his Socratic dialogue with Nick Jenkins, Toby Williamson notes that a danger of refuting humanism is that this posthumanism can be used to dehumanise people with cognitive impairment in a manner that inspires, permits and justifies mistreatment. Hence, this is not simply inconsequential intellectualised infighting. The potential ramifications of 'the critique of the critique' are significant (Ward & Sandberg 2023).

Intellectually, there is reason to be hopeful that our affinities will far outpace our frictions (though this is not to suggest that such frictions are not themselves valuably generative under the right conditions). It seems entirely plausible that productive resonances can be nurtured between, on the one hand, refuting human exceptionalism and, on the other hand, engaging with the politics of human difference. Indeed, the broader ontological turn across the social sciences and humanities may provide fertile terrain for taking critical dementia studies in several fruitful directions. To this end, Ann Lotherington's chapter concludes, for similar reasons, with a nod to the potential for feminist posthumanisms, in the manner popularised by Karen Barad (2003, 2007), to underpin new understandings of and responses to dementia. Traditionally, important scholarships have readily adapted to different theoretical imperatives. For instance, work on embodiment has attended to selfhood (Kontos 2004, 2005), selfhood and citizenship (Kontos, Miller & Kontos

2017), and citizenship and human rights (Kontos et al 2016). Moreover, it seems well-placed to engage with posthumanist predilections towards relational materialities. Indeed, commitments to materiality and citizenship are already being integrated to great effect (Lee & Bartlett 2021).

Conceptual developments such as material citizenship and embodied human rights are indicative of the generative resonances that can be cultivated by a dementia studies that is multi-disciplinary, multi-historied and multi-critical. The intellectual heritages of embodiment and human rights are highly divergent, particularly in their respective positioning of cognition. The traditions underpinning citizenship and new materialism have been in even greater, often explicit tension, catalysing wider disagreements between traditional critical theory and the ontological turn's complexification of materiality. The contemporary nebulousness of dementia studies effectively throws all of these histories into dialogue, provoking unpredictable collisions, conflicts and convergences that are the lifeblood of radical scholarships. To strictly appraise the criticality of such lifeblood in reference to a traditional definition of critical theory that is almost a century old seems to be somewhat at odds with the ethos of that tradition itself. Engagements at the margins of different disciplines and disciplinary traditions often seem particularly conducive to new ways of thinking. By 'margins' we mean the sense of positions that are not accepted or promulgated by the mainstream discipline. They used to often happen as conversations between people who still went outside to smoke at conferences, but those days have gone. This is a reminder that the cultural and architectural make up of institutions such as universities, and the forms of contact that they facilitate – e.g. chance coffee chats, Zoom meetings – are all important features in the continuation and transformation of dementia studies. As Mikhail Bahktin (1984: 252) observed: 'To be means to communicate dialogically. When dialogue ends, everything ends. Thus dialogue, by its very essence, cannot and must not come to an end'.

At a personal level, there is perhaps something important about the baton that gets passed on to new scholars in the field. Those of us who have been around for a long time have often had a gradual evolution in our thinking over time, which might not involve retracting things we said previously. Hence, beyond a certain point in anyone's career, it can become important to acknowledge that the new, and potentially unsettling, ideas are often coming from younger colleagues. If we continue hierarchically and resist this evolution, we risk ending up with a kind of concretised layer at the 'top' where things are unlikely to truly change because such change might be threatening. As an example, for people who have spent much of their career speaking about 'challenging behaviour', admitting that this is a pathologising concept could be existentially uprooting. Hence, there is something of a (inter) personal need for criticality if dementia studies is to continue to thrive.

Conclusion

In retrospect, critical dementia studies could be said to be defined by a loosely shared disposition towards treating dementia as a political category, which is achieved through de-normalising, de-naturalising and de-essentialising dementia.

From this perspective, quite a lot of the dementia studies canon is critical, or at least critical-leaning in its sensibilities, because this politicisation is a major portion of the work done by even the most rudimentary critiques of mainstream approaches to dementia, be they (bio)medical, heteronormative or humanist. The critical implication of this positioning of dementia as a political category is that its associated politics are fertile for transformation. If dementia is a political entity, then we can question it, resist it and agitate for change. This is perhaps as close to a definitive critical history of dementia studies as one can hope to achieve, recognising our place within a longstanding collection of agitations towards the politics of dementia. Mainstream treatments of dementia have long been troubling to dementia studies scholars, and in response, those scholars have long troubled dementia. For this reason, dementia studies as a constellation of social scientific and humanities scholarships has arguably long been an inherently multi-critical tradition.

References

Ballenger, J. F. (2017). Framing confusion: Dementia, society, and history. *AMA Journal of Ethics*, 19(7), 713–719.

Barad, K. (2003). Posthumanist performativity: Toward an understanding of how matter comes to matter. *Signs: Journal of Women in Culture and Society*, 28(3), 801–831.

Barad, K. (2007). *Meeting the Universe Halfway: Quantum Physics and the Entanglement of Matter and Meaning*. Durham: Duke University Press.

Bartlett, R. & O'Connor, D. (2010). *Broadening the Dementia Debate: Towards Social Citizenship*. Bristol: Policy Press.

Buber, M. (1923 [1937]). *I and Thou* [translated by Smith, R. G.]. Edinburgh: T & T Clark.

Conrad, P. (1975). The discovery of hyperkinesis: Notes on the medicalization of deviant behavior. *Social Problems*, 23(1), 12–21.

Fletcher, J. R. (2021a). Destigmatising dementia: The dangers of felt stigma and benevolent othering. *Dementia*, 20(2), 417–426.

Fletcher, J. R. (2021b). Black knowledges matter: How the suppression of non-white understandings of dementia harms us all and how we can combat it. *Sociology of Health & Illness*, 43(8), 1818–1825.

Fuller, S. C. (1912). Alzheimer's disease (*Senium præcox*): The report of a case and review of published cases. *Journal of Nervous and Mental Disease*, 39, 440–455.

Harding N. M. & Palfrey, C. (1997). *The Social Construction of Dementia: Confused Professionals?* London: Jessica Kingsley.

Herrup, K. (2021). *How Not to Study a Disease: The Story of Alzheimer's*. Cambridge: MIT Press.

Horkheimer, M. (1972). *Critical Theory: Selected Essays* (Vol. 1). New York: Continuum.

How, A. (2017). *Critical Theory*. London: Bloomsbury Publishing.

Kitwood, T. M. (1997). *Dementia Reconsidered: The Person Comes First*. Buckingham: Open University Press.

Kontos, P. C. (2004). Ethnographic reflections on selfhood, embodiment and Alzheimer's disease. *Ageing & Society*, 24(6), 829–849.

Kontos, P. C. (2005). Embodied selfhood in Alzheimer's disease: Rethinking person-centred care. *Dementia*, 4(4), 553–570.

Kontos, P., Grigorovich, A., Kontos, A. P., & Miller, K. L. (2016). Citizenship, human rights, and dementia: Towards a new embodied relational ethic of sexuality. *Dementia*, 15(3), 315–329.

Kontos, P., Miller, K. L., & Kontos, A. P. (2017). Relational citizenship: Supporting embodied selfhood and relationality in dementia care. *Sociology of Health & Illness*, 39(2), 182–198.

Lee, K., & Bartlett, R. (2021). Material Citizenship: An ethnographic study exploring object–person relations in the context of people with dementia in care homes. *Sociology of Health & Illness*, 43(6), 1471–1485.

Lévi-Strauss, C. (1962 [1966]). *The Savage Mind*. Chicago: Chicago University Press.

Mead, G. H. (1934). *Mind, Self and Society*. Chicago: Chicago University Press.

Pinel, P. (1806). *A Treatise on Insanity*. Sheffield: Cadell and Davies.

Powell, T. (2019). *Dementia Reimagined: Building a Life of Joy and Dignity from Beginning to End*. New York: Avery.

Prainsack, B. (2014). 'Personhood and solidarity: What kind of personalized medicine do we want?' *Personalized Medicine*, 11(7): 651–657.

Rogers, C. R. (1946). Significant aspects of client-centered therapy. *American Psychologist*, 1(10), 415–422.

Rothschild, D., & Trainor, M. A. (1937). Pathologic changes in senile psychoses and their psychobiologic significance. *American Journal of Psychiatry*, 93(4), 757–788.

Ward, R. & Sandberg, L. J. (2023). *Critical Dementia Studies*. London: Routledge.

Index

Note: Page references in **bold** denote tables and with "n" endnotes.

For Product Safety Concerns and Information please contact our EU
representative GPSR@taylorandfrancis.com
Taylor & Francis Verlag GmbH, Kaufingerstraße 24, 80331 München, Germany

www.ingramcontent.com/pod-product-compliance
Lightning Source LLC
Chambersburg PA
CBHW060300220326
41598CB00027B/4184